THE DEPTH
of BIRTH

Andrea Boyd Cohen

Illustrations by
Amanda Greavette & Nikki Scioscia

Depth of Birth

ISBN: 978-1-7348396-0-9

Library of Congress Control Number: 2020906099

Cover images and design by Nikki Scioscia
Book Design by Andrea Boyd & ElfElm Publishing
Illustrations by Nikki Scioscia, Amanda Greavette, and Jacob Lohmann
Author photograph by Erin Adams www.erinadamsphotography.com

Printed by DiggyPOD, Inc., in the United States of America.

First printing edition 2020

Andrea Boyd
dreboyd@mac.com
www.satoribirths.com

10 9 8 7 6 5 4 3 2 1

For my mother and father,
Pamela Bertoli Boyd
and Carl Richard Boyd
For their lives, my life, my child's life, and their
infinite love, nurturing, gifts, and presence.
Thank you for everything.
I love you.

For my husband and son,
Jeffrey Daniel Cohen and Dove Satori Cohen
You enrich this world with who you are.
My heart bursts with joy.
I love you.
Thank you.

DISCLAIMER

The information provided in this book is designed to provide helpful information on the subjects discussed. This book is not meant for use to diagnose or treat any medical condition. The publisher and author are not responsible for any specific health or allergy needs that may require medical supervision. They are not liable for any damages or negative consequences from any treatment, action, application, or preparation, to any person reading or following the information in this book.

The author and publisher make no representations or warranties of any kind and assume no liabilities of any kind concerning the accuracy or completeness of the contents and expressly disclaim any implied warranties of merchantability or fitness of use for a particular purpose. Neither the author nor the publisher shall be held liable or responsible to any person or entity concerning any loss, incidental or consequential damages caused, or alleged to have been produced, directly or indirectly, by the information contained herein.

The publisher is not engaged to render any psychological, legal, or any other kind of professional advice. The content of this book is the sole expression of its author. Neither the publisher nor the individual author(s) shall be liable for any physical, psychological, emotional, financial, or commercial damages, including, but not limited to, special, incidental, consequential or other damages. Our views and rights are the same: You are responsible for your own choices, actions, and results. References are provided for informational purposes only and do not constitute endorsement of any websites or other sources. Readers should be aware that the website addresses listed in this book may change.

PREFACE

In December of 2010, my husband and I had traveled to Bali to my dear friend Michael Franti's home. He took us to a place called Bhumi Sehat and introduced us to a woman named Robin Lim. It is a birthing clinic that provides women a safe and sacred atmosphere to give birth. Women who may not be able to afford other care, who want to be around other women, who want to have a gentle birthing environment. As we walked through the clinic, she showed us the birthing tubs and spoke about the offerings such as yoga, cranial-sacral therapy, prenatal vitamins, and herbal tea. She talked about how when the baby is born, she and the other midwives softly sing a mantra or prayer into their ear. She told us that if a woman birthed in the local hospital and could not afford the bill she was not allowed to take the baby home until it had been paid. I later realized the stories she told were the seeds planted in me to become an advocate for gentle births. It ignited in me the desire that women have a supportive and loving pregnancy and birthing experience, and that babies are born in an environment where it is considered a most sacred event. I remember saying to Robin, "If I ever have a baby, I would want you to be my midwife." She encouraged me to do so.

In February 2015, I found out that I was pregnant, and had all day long "morning sickness" for the next three months or so. I rested and read, educating myself about midwifery, the umbilical cord, birthing positions, etc. I watched the film about Ina May Gaskin, the well-known midwife from The Farm. I realized how little I had known about birth, and felt that it was a reasonably important part of life to discover!

Meanwhile, my friend Vikki had begun a non-for-profit, commercial-free radio station, and was looking for content that would be enlightening to the listener. I shared with her that I wanted to offer a show, but hadn't decided what the content would be. Then one night, a wave of creativity came through me and out poured the idea to create a show about birth. To share what I was learning, and to interview midwives, doulas, doctors, mothers, fathers, children. I typed out topic ideas, subtopics, chose songs to enhance the show, and at the end, had about 17 shows ready to be written and recorded. It would be called "The Depth of Birth."

I offered the shows as a way to explore and discuss elements of birth that go unspoken about, or unchallenged, or are unknown, considered strange, etc.

Those who heard the shows exclaimed to me that they were learning. As a yoga teacher, I am often asked by newly pregnant women, "What books do you recommend?" I found myself wanting to be able to hand them a copy of the information found in the radio shows and therefore decided, The Depth of Birth shall become a book! So here in your hands is the fruit of those seeds planted years ago, from someone who at many points in life did not even want to have children, who is known to take the road less traveled, and who likes to look deeply into the nature of our nature and existence.

In birthing my son, October of 2015, after hours of contractions, bouts of pain from his head pressing my sciatic nerve, and time in the birthing pool, I began sobbing. Tears were pouring from me for quite a while, and I later came to realize that they were tears not only for myself, for my baby, but all the women in the world; those who have children, those who want children, those who do not, those who have not been able to get pregnant easily or at all, single mothers, impoverished mothers, abused women, violated and manipulated women and young girls, women who have lost their children in childbirth, or during the pregnancy, women who have been raped, women who for whatever reason had an abortion, women with abusive partners, women with postpartum depression, women who experience shame or degradation, women who feel unsupported, unempowered, teenage mothers, and the list goes on…

It is time in our culture, and in the world, to embrace the womb, the mother, the divine feminine, the creatress in the universe. It is time to treat birth as a sacred event. To treat the mother as light, love, vessel, rather than a patient. She is not sick. She is bringing forth a soul encased in a body into the realm we share. No one is "delivering" the baby for her. She is an active participant. She is birthing this being. She is capable, supple, powerful, uniquely designed to do so. It has been going on for thousands of years. Like other animals, who go into private, low-lit spaces, and follow their intuition, follow their breath, follow the rhythm of pulsation, life, baby, we too can take back birth. A woman's intuition is strong. Her inner wisdom is vast. If the inner voice is lost, the natural inclination is also lost. Our ancestors, the ancient ones, are cheering for us to return to that place where fear does not dominate; where we trust our bodies and go back to the origin of all—LOVE.

October 15, 2016

Tulum, Mexico

ᔕ

INFORMATION IN THIS BOOK

I am determined to contribute to a world that embraces gentle and sacred births, empowered and satisfied mothers, respectful and individualized care, and a population that understands the risks and detriment of popular practices in the current-day environment. In terms of mother's rights, it is essential that women be offered more self-determination, more information, more options, and less fear during pregnancy, labor, and birth. As for babies, their delicacy, sensitivity, and vibrancy must be protected, as they transition through phases in the womb, and out into the world. Consideration for them as intelligent individuals may help curb excessive: ultrasound testing, augmentation to rush them out when unnecessary, epidural narcotics to dull labor sensations, removal of baby from mother's arms soon after birth, cutting of the genitals, painful shots, rough handling of the newborn, etc.

What I provide in this book is some information that will be a helpful start in learning about these topics in regards to how new life is ushered into the world. I intended to create a book that would inspire you to learn even more beyond what is on these pages. To be comprehensive, this book would have to be volumes and volumes. Because this book will be printed, the statistics found within may be outdated, but still relevant.

There are so many others who seek, ask, and realize, and who have provided me with excellent content in various ways for this book. I have spent countless hours researching, reading, interviewing people, watching films, talking to mothers, finding out policies, experiencing birth firsthand, pondering, questioning, and having realizations of my own. Additionally, being a doula has been incredibly illuminating.

The list below are some superb resources that were helpful in providing statistics and information. The books, films, and websites in the back of the book were also utilized. I offer great appreciation to those who have done studies, researched, and written on these topics, so that I too can share them.

- Birth Monopoly & Cristen Pascucci
- Midwifery Today
- The National Center for Biotechnology Information
- American College of Obstetrics and Gynecology
- Doulas of North America
- Spinning Babies
- Improving Birth
- World Health Organization
- American Pregnancy
- Psychology Today
- Citizens for Midwifery
- Science and Sensibility
- Chris Kresser
- Robin Lim, CPM (Bhumi Sehat)
- Dr. Sarah J Buckley
- Kelly Winder (BellyBelly, Australia)
- Genevieve Howland (Mama Natural)
- Rebecca Dekker, PhD, RN (Evidence Based Birth)
- Kelly Bonyata, BS, International Board Certified Lactation Consultant (kellymom)

CONTENTS

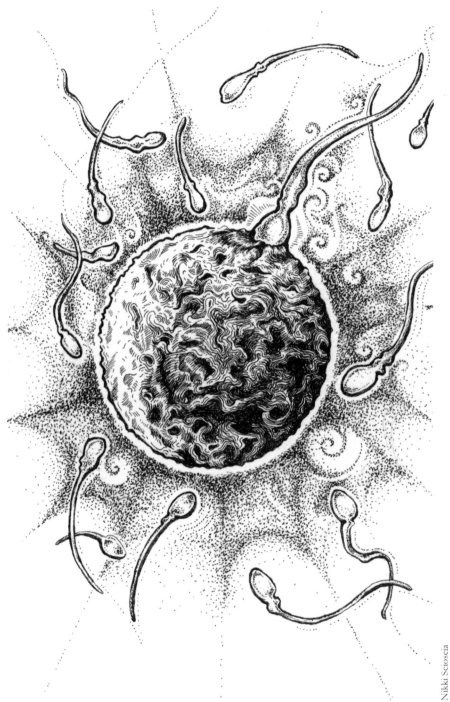

CHAPTER 1: PREGNANCY

*"Pay attention to the pregnant woman! There
is no one as important as she!"*
- CHAGGA SAYING, UGANDA

*"It seems that many health professionals involved in
antenatal care have not realized that one of their roles should
be to protect the emotional state of pregnant women."*
- MICHAEL ODENT, M.D.

*"The knowledge about how to give birth is born within every
woman: women do not need to be taught how to give birth but
rather to have more trust and faith in their own body knowledge."*
- BIRTHWORKS

SOME WOMEN TAKE A pregnancy test, hoping it says no, while others take a test praying it says yes. I have experienced both hopes and feelings. Seeing the sign on a stick, whether positive or negative, is a monumental occasion. The woman may feel elated, shocked, full of despair, overwhelmed, overjoyed, and perhaps many of those emotions at once. Pregnancy involves a myriad of hormones, decisions, bodily changes, and growth—both physically, mentally, and spiritually. It is miraculous and abundant. The feeling of someone moving around inside, kicking, and hiccupping is mind-boggling, and the experience and sheer reality of growing another human being will never cease amazing me.

CONCEPTION (adapted from health.howstuffworks.com)
A man releases millions of sperm with each ejaculation. Inside the woman's body, these sperm swim fast to find the egg. If one reaches the egg and penetrates it, fertilization occurs. Things begin progressing rapidly inside the mother's womb. The sperm and egg merge to form a little single-celled organism called a zygote, which consists of the 23 chromosomes from the

man's sperm and the 23 chromosomes from the female's egg. These chromosomes will determine the baby's hair color, eye color, and whether the baby will be a boy or a girl.

Soon after fertilization, the zygote travels through the fallopian tubes to the uterus. During the journey, the zygote divides, and within 72 hours, it will have gone from one cell to eight cells. The zygote divides until it contains about 100 cells. Then it becomes known as a blastocyst. The inner group of cells will form the embryo. The outer group of cells forms the placenta, which will provide nourishment.

Three weeks into the pregnancy, the blastocyst implants itself into the mother's uterine wall and releases human chorionic gonadotropin (hCG), a hormone produced only during pregnancy. This occurs only a few days after conception. Home pregnancy tests measure hCG in urine, while a test in the doctor's office will identify hCG in a blood sample. The blood test can pick up miniscule amounts of the hormone and identify pregnancy earlier than a home pregnancy test. Still, most home tests are 97 to 99% accurate if taken correctly. The midwife or doctor will begin counting the 40 weeks of pregnancy from the start of the last period, although conception normally occurs about two weeks after that. {Which is why most woman will give birth AFTER their "due date"!}

By the fifth week of the pregnancy, the brain, spinal cord, heart, and other organs begin to form. The embryo is now made up of three layers: the ectoderm, mesoderm, and endoderm. Every organ and tissue will develop out of these three layers. The ectoderm will form the nervous system and backbone; the mesoderm will form the heart and circulatory system; and the endoderm will form the lungs, gastrointestinal tract, thyroid, liver and pancreas. The umbilical cord and placenta have begun to form, which will deliver nutrients to, and remove wastes from, the growing embryo.

FIRST TRIMESTER (weeks 1–12)
Although the embryo is the size of a sesame seed, the mother-to-be will likely start feeling the first twinges of pregnancy. Morning sickness, frequent urination, sleepiness, and food cravings or aversions are all common. The breasts may swell and become tender. At this point in pregnancy, the woman will have her first prenatal visit with a midwife or obstetrician. The mother

should be especially careful in the first trimester, during the formation of the delicate organs; avoiding alcohol, certain medications, caffeine, and smoking, taking prenatal vitamins containing folic acid with a healthy diet and regular exercise.

SECOND TRIMESTER (weeks 13–27)

For many women, the second trimester is a definite improvement. As the nausea recedes and exhaustion abates, energy and appetite return. Though the fetus is just a few inches long, the belly is growing. Mammary ducts inside the mother's breasts prepare to produce milk. During this trimester, the breasts will start to produce a yellowish, nutrient-rich substance called colostrum, which will feed the baby during the first few days of life.

At week 20—halfway through the pregnancy—the fetus is about six inches long and weighs about 10 ounces. Its digestive system produces meconium, a black, tar-like substance that will make up its first few bowel movements. The fetus is coated in a white greasy substance called vernix caseosa, which will protect its skin from the amniotic fluid in utero. The fetus will swallow and "breathe" amniotic fluid to train its digestive system and lungs. Its lungs produce a substance called surfactant, which will enable the air sacs to inflate for breathing once it is born.

THIRD TRIMESTER (weeks 28–birth)

During the next 12 weeks, the fetus will finish its development and prepare for the difficult birth process. It is now about 15 inches long and weighs between two and three pounds. The eyes are a definite color (although they may change after it is born) and are fringed with lashes. The body is rounding out as fat deposits under the skin. This fat will help regulate his/her body temperature once born. The brain is becoming larger and more defined, and skull growing to accommodate it. If the fetus is a boy, his testicles are descending into his scrotum. If a girl, her clitoris is developed.

As the mother's belly swells, she may be in more discomfort, especially near the end of her pregnancy. The pressure of the growing uterus on the diaphragm may also make her feel short of breath. It can press down on nerves, causing pain in her lower back and legs, and constrict her bladder, making her run to the bathroom constantly. Many women feel tired and have difficulty sleeping because of their increasing girth.

BIRTH

Once her cervix is dilated entirely to 10 cm, the mother's body is ready to start pushing. The combined force of uterine contractions and the mother's meeting of the pressure, move the baby down the birth canal. Eventually, the baby's head will descend to the mother's perineum (the tissue that stretches between the vagina and rectum). Pressure on the perineum can feel like burning or stinging when the baby "crowns," or when the widest part of its head becomes visible.

FUN FACT

Did you know that the longest female human pregnancy on record is 375 days long?

HAVE A GLORIOUS PREGNANCY!

You are growing a human being inside of your body. WOW! Keep the feeling of this magical event going, with all of the hills and valleys that pregnancy might bring, to stay well physically, emotionally, and mentally.

WALKING

My friend suggested to me to walk 5 miles a day, to keep feeling strong and fit. I tried as best I could, and it did. Some days my intuition would kick in, saying, "Turn around here," and I would walk home short of 5 miles, but the goal gave me incentive to do whatever amount that I could. I am eternally grateful because my body felt great up until and throughout labor and birthing. Keep your legs active, mamas!

SWIMMING

As baby grows and belly expands, you will want to feel weightlessness now and again. Swimming can do this. Hop into an ocean, lake, river, pool, bathtub, and enjoy the buoyancy. Make sure not to get into strong currents or rocky areas, staying safe.

YOGA (asanas, exercises, meditation, mantras, music)
Find a prenatal class, or if it's not available in person, on the Internet. Yoga classes will stretch your body to stay supple and tension-free, as well as focused, energetic, relaxed, and able to breathe deeply. Most importantly, you will become more acquainted with your breath. With deep breathing, you can relax, slow the heart rate, and open. If you learn to control and harness your breath, you learn to control your endorphins, enliven the power of your birthing instincts, and stay calm throughout labor and birthing. You will also meet other mothers in various stages of pregnancy and make connections and friends.

HYDRATION
Drink, drink, drink! Have water near you at all times. Pick a large cup, or thermos, & take it everywhere. Tell your partner that wherever you are, to please bring you water/make sure you have some. Continue this after birth, to stay hydrated, and keep breast milk flowing.

RED RASPBERRY LEAF TEA
Raspberry leaf is the leaf of the raspberry plant. It is naturally high in magnesium, potassium, iron, Vitamin C, and b-vitamins, which make it helpful for nausea, leg cramps, and improving sleep during pregnancy. The specific combination of nutrients makes it extremely beneficial for the female reproductive system. It strengthens the uterus and pelvic muscles, which some midwives say leads to shorter and easier labors. The tannins in raspberry leaf give it astringent properties, which make it soothing both internally and externally. Although red raspberry leaf is an herb with centuries of safe use behind it and little cause for concern, if a mother is prone to miscarriages, she may want to avoid it until the third trimester. Mountain Rose Herbs is an organic, high-quality supplier.

PRENATAL VITAMINS
Go with whole foods-based and organic. You may have to try a couple of brands, in case one particular brand makes you feel queasy. Here are some great ones, which can be found online and in stores: Garden of Life "My

Kind," New Chapter "Perfect Prenatal," MegaFood "Baby & Me," Rainbow Light "Prenatal One," Solaray "Once Daily Prenatal."

NOURISHING VEGETARIAN/VEGAN FOOD

(organic if available): Fruits, veggies, grains, legumes, oils, nuts, noodles, potatoes, tempeh, tofu, soups, breads, nut butters, animal meat alternatives, salads…

POSITIVITY

Offer yourself and other pregnant women optimism, empowerment, and support. People will have their opinions about your decisions. Stay upbeat and keep negativity away. For example, someone asks you where you plan to birth, and you say, "At the birth center." If they say, "You should be in a hospital," or tell you stories full of fear or negativity, say, "Thank you, but I would rather not hear that at this moment." Or excuse yourself to the bathroom before they get far along—you likely have to pee anyway!

There seems to be this idea that pregnant women are supposed to be miserable, complaining, having problems, and that the birth is supposed to be painful. FORGET THAT! You have a miracle occurring inside of your body, and a cocktail of hormones mixing. Another soul is living in your womb! As a pregnant woman, change this cultural stigma and celebrate with optimism. Make a promise to your baby (who can hear you, by the way) to not complain. When around other pregnant mamas, share your optimism and be optimistic about their pregnancy and birth too. Revel in the changes of the body, the glowing skin, the lustrous hair, and remember how beautiful you are. Walk tall and proud to be carrying another human being inside of your body!

CHALLENGES THAT MAY ARISE

NAUSEA/VOMITING

Eat little and often. When your stomach is empty, the acids have nothing to feast on but your stomach lining, compounding nausea. On the other hand, overeating can overtax the digestive system and lead to queasiness. Keeping a little bit full all day and night is the best defense against "morning/all day sickness." Plain foods such as potatoes, pasta, rice, and dry crackers are often easier to stomach. Figure out which foods make your symptoms worse. A lot is going on in there, so take deep breaths and eat what you can keep down (for me it was green apples, mashed potatoes, and tofu scramble). Stay hydrated.

SMELLS

Your sense of smell is heightened. You may be disgusted by certain smells, like cigarette smoke, the grocery store, dead fish, coffee, your husband's shampoo, maybe even your husband! Share with those around you what triggers it. I told my husband if he wanted coffee, he had to buy it and drink it down the road somewhere.

FATIGUE

Your body is working extra hard. You are growing a human being inside of you. So, fatigue is natural and will prepare you for the combination of less sleep and beautiful daily play/work of being a parent. Get plenty of sleep. Rest when you need to. Take time off of work.

VARICOSE VEINS

As your uterus grows, it puts pressure on the large vein on the right side of your body (inferior vena cava), which in turn increases pressure in the leg veins. Hormonal changes can also lead to varicose veins as increased progestin levels can dilate or open the veins. Varicose veins typically diminish within three months to a year after giving birth. The following can help prevent/reduce them:

- Sit sideways with one shoulder towards the wall, getting buttocks as close to the wall as you can. Place hands alongside you and lie down on your back, bringing the legs up the wall slowly and gently. Slide a folded firm blanket underneath the lower back/sacrum. This position also helps with circulation, relaxation, and energy.
- Elevate your legs when you sit
- Keep fit with walking, swimming, and yoga
- Sleep on your left side
- Don't strain
- Drink lots of water

STRETCH MARKS

Rub shea butter on your body, especially the breasts to keep them moisturized, stimulated, and prepare them for breastfeeding. Take cold showers to improve metabolism, immunity, and circulation, increase endorphins, and ease stress. It is invigorating, boosting your energy and mood. Start slow by lowering the water temperature for a couple of minutes. Deep breathing helps.

HEMORRHOIDS

Hemorrhoids are swollen veins in the lowest part of your rectum and anus, also called piles. Sometimes the walls of these blood vessels stretch so thin that the veins bulge and get irritated, especially when you defecate. External hemorrhoids are small lumps outside of the rectum, which can be painful and itchy. Symptoms include rectal bleeding, itching, burning and pain or pressure, a bulge on the anus, bright red blood on toilet paper. During pregnancy, the uterus and blood volume increases, placing more pressure on the veins that run through the anus, causing them to swell. They most often appear during the third trimester. They may also develop postpartum as a result of pushing during labor.

Or they could come from:
- Pushing during bowel movements
- Straining when doing something physically hard/lifting something heavy
- Prolonged standing or sitting

THESE MAY HELP RELIEVE/REMEDY:
- Place baking soda (wet or dry) on the area to reduce itching
- Take a warm bath with baking soda in the water
- Use cold witch hazel on a cotton ball to reduce bleeding
- Place an ice cube in a small cotton napkin and hold directly on the lump(s)
- A half a cup of radish juice consumed twice daily or an application of shredded radish directly on the lump(s)
- Mango seed powder is known to relieve swelling, pain, and itching sensation (1–2 teaspoons twice a day)

- Horse Chestnuts or Aesculus hippocastanum contain a saponin compound called aescin. Aescin is an anti-inflammatory, eases inflammation and strengthens blood vessels.
- Legs up the wall (see yoga section above)
- Turmeric has anti-inflammatory, antibacterial, antiseptic, antioxidant, and anti-allergic properties. It is effective both topically and internally.

Try the following to prevent constipation:
- Eat lots of fiber
- Drink plenty of water
- Do not delay going to the bathroom
- Eat plenty of fruits and vegetables
- Avoid sitting for long periods
- Avoid heavy lifting
- Wear loose underwear and cotton clothing (most breathable fabric)

SWELLING

Edema in the hands, feet, and ankles is common (especially during the heat of summer). During pregnancy, the volume of blood in a woman's body increases by a whopping 50% to help support the uterus. Accordingly, the amount of blood pumped by the heart increases as well. Swimming, keeping legs uncrossed, massage, propping feet, and legs up the wall are helpful.

BACKACHE

Stretching, yoga, good posture, and awareness of weight distribution in the feet are useful in preventing or relieving backache. Make sure you are standing and walking on the full foot, not only on the heels. There is a tendency to lean back when pregnant, due to the growing weight/belly on the front body.

TROUBLE SLEEPING

You may need to enlist the assistance of multiple pillows, or for some women, a body pillow, to get comfortable. A pillow between the legs or under the knees can be helpful. Most mothers instinctively sleep on their sides. Because your liver is on the right side of your abdomen, lying on your left side helps keep the uterus off that large organ. Sleeping on the left side improves circulation to the heart and allows for the best blood flow to the fetus, uterus, and kidneys. But sleeping on the right side is also fine, and better than on your stomach or back. When you lie on your back, the weight of your uterus can compress a major blood vessel called the vena cava, disrupting blood flow to the baby and possibly leaving you nauseated, dizzy, and/or short of breath.

PUPP RASH

PUPP stands for Pruritic Urticarial Papules and Plaques, and is a skin condition that can arrive in pregnancy. Small, red, itchy bumps on the skin, which usually begin in the abdominal area and spread outward. Often labor induction will be recommended to alleviate symptoms; however, induction carries its risks and complications and is not considered effective at stopping PUPPS. PUPPS can also develop after delivery, so again, induction is not a surefire remedy.

During pregnancy some preventative measures to take: wear loose-fitting, lightweight cotton shirts, avoid using toxic and irritating chemicals in laundry detergents, soaps, fragrances, lotions, shampoos, makeup, deodorant, etc. Use natural ingredients.

THESE MAY HELP ALLEVIATE ITCHING/DISCOMFORT

Dandelion Root & Nettle Tea: An overtaxed liver is a possible contributor to PUPPS, so anything to support the liver will help. Dandelion root and nettle are liver and blood purifiers traditionally used by midwives and herbalists as an effective remedy. Dandelion root supports the liver while nettles are a natural antihistamine and anti-inflammatory agent. Nettles are also used during pregnancy to help with anemia because it raises iron levels.

Recipe: Steep one tea bag of dandelion root or one tsp. of loose tea in 1 cup of boiling water for at least 10 minutes and up to 1 hour. Do the same with nettle leaf. Add them together.

*Note: Dandelion root capsules and sulfur tablets are also popular cures.

Anti-Inflammatory Herbs: Chamomile, Calendula and Chinese Skullcap can reduce skin inflammation when applied topically. Adding these herbs (in extract form) to soothing aloe vera, witch hazel, or sesame oil can alleviate the hot and irritating sensation that the rash can bring.

Recipe: Rub the herbal infused aloe/lotion/oil onto the abdomen, 3X a day.

Oatmeal Bath: Soaking in an oatmeal bath can relieve the itchiness, soothe and moisturize the skin, and can be done several times a day. You can also make a strong tea with the herbs mentioned above and add to the bath.

Recipe: Place 1 cup of rolled oats and 1 cup of organic chamomile loose tea into some cheesecloth or an old t-shirt and secure tightly with a rubber band. Place in tub and soak for at least 20 minutes. Occasionally squeeze the oats to release their milky liquid.

Pine Tar Soap: Use up to 4X a day on rash.

Coconut or Sesame Oil: Use a high-quality organic brand. Apply to area.

Vegetable & Fruit Juices: (Carrots, Beets, Cucumbers, Celery, Fennel, Peppers, Ginger, Apples, Lemons, Oranges, Pineapple) & Black Cherry Juice. Drink as often as you desire.

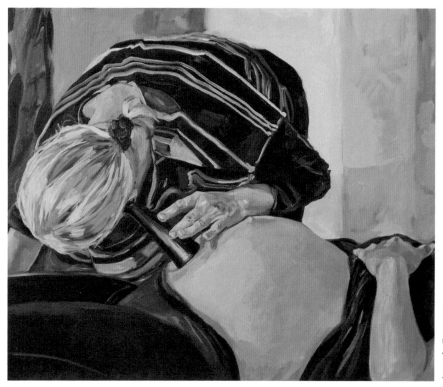

Amanda Greavette

CHAPTER 2:
MIDWIVES & MIDWIFERY

"Midwives see birth as a miracle and only mess with it if there's a problem; doctors see birth as a problem and if they don't mess with it, it's a miracle!"

- BARBARA HARPER
Gentle Birth Choices

"Every midwife knows that not until a mother's womb softens from the pain of labor will a way unfold and the infant find that opening to be born. Oh friend! There is treasure in your heart. It is heavy with child. Listen. All the awakened ones, like trusted midwives are saying, 'Welcome this pain. It opens the dark passage of Grace."

-RUMI

"Experiences have clearly shown that an approach which 'de-medicalizes' birth, restores dignity and humanity to the process of childbirth, and returns control to the mother, is also the safest approach."

- MICHEL ODENT, MD

THE DAY I FOUND out I was pregnant, I called around to local midwives to find the right match. When the second one arrived at our apartment door, my husband and I both knew she was the one. She was laidback, confident, soft-spoken, and receptive. She answered all of my questions patiently and thoroughly. Our meetings were in our living room, usually over shared rooibos tea and berries. She was gentle, caring, kind, and fearless. Had my husband not caught our baby when he arrived outside, she was someone I would want as the first touch for my child. The precious and fragile newborn should be treated with gentle, loving hands.

WHAT IS A MIDWIFE?

Midwives are trained professionals with expertise and skills in supporting women to maintain healthy pregnancies and experience optimal births and postpartum recoveries. Midwives provide women with individualized care uniquely suited to their physical, mental, emotional, spiritual, and cultural needs. When the care required is outside of the midwife's scope of practice or expertise-such as high risks pregnancies or preexisting health issues—she refers the mother-to-be to other healthcare providers for additional consultation or care. Midwives believe that birth is a natural physiological process that should be inherently trusted. Midwifery is a woman-centered empowering model of maternity care utilized in all countries of the world with the best maternal and infant outcomes, such as The Netherlands, Canada, and the United Kingdom.

A comprehensive look into the work and life of midwives was explored the Pulitzer Prize-winning book, *A Midwife's Tale: The Life of Martha Ballard*, written by Laurel Thatcher Ulrich. Ulrich chronicled her career as a midwife from when she began in 1785, to when she caught her last of 996 babies in 1812.

PATHS OF MIDWIFERY

Nurse-midwives are educated and licensed as nurses first, before completing additional education in midwifery. They receive certification from the American Midwifery Certification Board (AMCB) and are known as Certified Nurse-Midwives (CNMs). CNMs are licensed to practice in all 50 states. They are usually licensed in individual states as Nurse Practitioners (NPs). The American College of Nurse-Midwives (ACNM) is the professional association representing CNMs and Certified Midwives (CMs) in the United States.

Direct-entry midwives are educated or trained as midwives without having to become nurses first. They may be Certified Professional Midwives (CPMs) or Certified Midwives (CMs). CPMs receive certification by the North American Registry of Midwives (NARM). The legal status and requirements for direct-entry (non-nurse) midwives vary from state-to-state. They are licensed in individual states as Licensed Midwives (LMs) or Registered Midwives (RMs). The Midwives Alliance of North America tracks the laws and regulations in each state for direct-entry midwives.

Women who learned the practice of midwifery from their mothers, grandmothers, etc. are called "granny midwives." For many poor and rural women, particularly in the South, granny midwives were lifesavers. "Lay midwives" refer to uncertified or unlicensed midwives, who were trained in their communities by an informal education, apprenticing with a practicing midwife and self-study.

In 2014, midwives attended 332,107 births, or 8.3% of babies born in the U.S. What is the most midwife-friendly state? New Mexico-where midwives bring 24% of all babies in that state. In countries like the Denmark and Sweden the entire birth process is managed by midwives. Men midwives exist too.

A TIMELINE OF MIDWIFERY HERSTORY

For centuries, women attended women during childbirth. Midwives were tapped into the wisdom of sense experience, observation, perception, and evidence, and knew their craft well. Birth took place at home or in a birthing hut, in the baby's natural time, with the mother surrounded by a network of intuitive women trained through generations of organic, sensitive, nourishing and spiritual birthing practices. These women attendants were skilled in assisting the mother by providing soothing comfort measures and nourishment. They patiently waited for nature to take its course without undue interference with the normal process of labor and birth.

During the 17th and 18th centuries, only when complications arose during childbirth did women turn to the barber-surgeons who emerged during the Renaissance in Western Europe. Whereas women in the countryside were generally healthy and well equipped to birth babies, women in newly developed cities were prone to disease and thus to complications in birth. In these cases, the barber-surgeons with their suitable tools were called upon to extract the baby from a mother's deformed pelvis (from rickets, due to malnourishment), the only alternative for sparing the mother from death. These barber-surgeons, who formed guilds to house their similar vocations, saw the profit in aiding midwives during childbirth and in perfecting tools to do so. In 1588, Peter Chamberlen invented the obstetric forceps, laying the foundation for surgical instruments and medical interventions during birth.

Up until the 19th century, midwifery was still an organic field of its own, relatively untouched by outside medical practices. As time passed and research in the field of medicine progressed, labor and birthing led to the medical specialty of obstetrics. While midwifery was, by and large, a female profession, men dominated the medical field. Male physicians received more formal education except in the physiological female process of giving birth. Obstetricians began implementing techniques that, although intended to minimize women's suffering during birth, were not necessarily sensitive to the potential long-term effects such maneuvers had on women's psyche and reproductive organs.

Formal education created a significant divide between the fields of obstetrics and midwifery. Midwives' expertise wasn't as recognized, and they sought out higher education to remain on level with obstetrics but experienced much pushback. The gap grew wider once physicians introduced anesthesia to the birthing process at the end of the 19th century. Also introduced, implemented, and encouraged, as outlined in Dr. Joseph B. DeLee's article, "The Prophylactic Forceps Operation" (American Journal of Obstetrics and Gynecology, 1920), were forceps, narcotics, episiotomy, and Pitocin, all conducted only at a hospital, and obstetricians adopted the consistent use of these.

In Europe, schools for midwives came to be, and midwives and obstetricians were able to work in relative conjunction with each other. Midwives tended to normal births, while physicians handled births with complications. In the United States, though midwifery was generally supported by public health care reform, physicians worked against midwifery education, pushing to move all births from homes to hospitals. At the beginning of the 20th century, over 90% of births occurred at home; by 1950, over 90% occurred in the hospital. This change was partially due to anesthesia being almost universally used during childbirth by the 1920s. The shift to the hospital did not decrease the mortality rates for mothers. It wasn't until 1935, when antibiotics and blood transfusions became part of the standard, that mortality rates became drastically reduced. In the 1960s and 1970s, there was a rise in advocacy for natural childbirth and women's decision-making, led by the Women's Movement, but routine interventions remain prevalent to this day.

Midwives have comparatively bridged the gap between midwifery and obstetrics through formal education. But the practice of midwifery is in jeopardy due to: a lack of awareness, lack of information and accessibility of care to mothers, rising malpractice insurance costs, women's trust in technology, and renewed efforts to prevent autonomous midwifery by professional medical associations and state regulators. Midwives continue to fight for their place in the practice of childbirth.

In 1846, the Hungairan Dr. Ignaz Semmelweiss collected data to figure out why so many women in maternity wards were dying from puerperal fever, commonly known as childbed fever. He studied two wards: one staffed by all male doctors and medical students and another staffed by female midwives. The death rate was 5 times higher in the doctor's ward. Doctors did autopsies, and cadaverous particles remained on their hands from the corpses they dissected, so he ordered them to clean their hands with chlorine to disinfect, and the rate of childbed fever fell dramatically.

MIDWIFERY LINEAGE

These women are legendary to the towns they lived and to midwives around the world.

MARY BRECKINRIDGE (Hyden, Kentucky, 1881–1965)

After the death of both her children at an early age, she dedicated her life to improving the health of women and children and became a registered nurse in 1910. After meeting nurse-midwives in France and London, she decided to work in this field. She saw that women lacked prenatal care. In 1925, she founded the Frontier Nursing Service (FNS), with staff composed of nurse-midwives trained in England, who traveled on horseback and foot to provide quality care in the clients' homes. No one was denied care, and maternal and infant mortality rates decreased dramatically in this area. FNS staff started the first American school of midwifery in New York, and the American Association of Nurse-Midwives, who recognize her as "the first to bring nurse-midwifery to the United States." In 1982, she was inducted into the American Nurses Association's Hall of Fame.

MAUDE E. CALLEN (Pineville, South Carolina, USA, 1898–1990)
Nurse Maude was born in Florida, had twelve sisters, was orphaned at the age of six, and brought up in the home of her uncle, a physician in Tallahassee. Callen devoted her life to nursing in a poverty-stricken area, operating a clinic out of her home. In conditions with no electricity, roads, or cars, and through mud, woods, and creeks, she arrived to mothers in the middle of the night, ushering in about 800 babies in her 62 years of practice. She trained midwives in her community and throughout the county, teaching proper methods in prenatal care, labor support, baby delivery, and handling of newborns. She was honored with the Alexis de Tocqueville Society Award for 60 years of service to her community. In 1989, the Medical University of South Carolina gave her an honorary degree, and their College of Nursing created a scholarship in her name. In December of 1951, *Life* magazine published a lengthy photographic essay of Callen's work by photojournalist W. Eugene Smith. Smith spent weeks with her, and later said, "she was the most completely fulfilled person I have ever known."

MARY FRANCIS HILL COLEY (Albany, Georgia, 1900–1966)
In over 30 years "Miss Mary" caught more than 3,000 babies in five counties in Georgia. She was known for her tireless work ethic and willingness to serve both black and white mothers in the segregated South. Her care of new families extended beyond the baby's arrival. She would visit for days after the birth to cook, clean, and wash clothes. She knew her work was a spiritual calling, and let nothing keep her from mothers who needed her. In 1952, documentarian George Stoney filmed a movie produced by the Georgia Health Department as an instructional film, following Coley as she went about her work. *All My Babies: A Midwife's Own Story* follows her through the births of two babies and is used in training midwives all over the world. The film was critically acclaimed and selected by the Library of Congress for placement on the National Film Registry as "a culturally, historically and artistically significant work."

MARGARET CHARLES SMITH (Greene County, Alabama, 1906–2004)
Smith unexpectedly began her career as a midwife when she was five years old and was asked to stay with a laboring mother while the father went for

the midwife. Before they returned, Smith caught the baby! Smith often had to make her way through fields and wade through water before catching up to four babies a night. The mothers she attended were often malnourished and overworked. She delivered twins, breech babies, and premature babies. Some mothers could not afford to pay her anything, and sometimes she received produce or $5–$10 in return. In 1976, Alabama passed a law outlawing midwives. Smith and about 150 other black traditional midwives were told they would be jailed if they continued to work as midwives, but she continued. In 1983, she became the first black American to be given the keys to her hometown of Eutaw, Alabama, and honored at the first Black Women's Health Project in Atlanta, Georgia. In 1996, she co-authored a book with Linda Janet Holmes called *Listen to Me Good: The Life Story of an Alabama Midwife*.

FAMOUS MODERN DAY MIDWIVES

INA MAY GASKIN (1940-present)

Ina May Gaskin, MA, CPM, PhD (Hon.), a midwife for over 40 years, is founder and director of The Farm Midwifery Center, a birthing community near Summertown, Tennessee, founded in 1971. The Farm is noted for its low rates of intervention, morbidity and mortality despite the inclusion of many vaginally delivered breeches, twins, vaginal births after cesareans, and grand multiparas (mothers who have birthed 5+ times). Gaskin has lectured all over the world at midwifery conferences and medical schools, to students and faculty. Her promotion of an extremely effective method for dealing with one of the most-feared birth complications, shoulder dystocia, has become known as The Gaskin Maneuver and is the first obstetrical procedure to be named for a midwife. It originated in Guatemala. Her expertise on breech deliveries has sparked reconsideration in regards to the policy of automatically performing cesarean for breech babies. She has received many awards, including the Right Livelihood Award (also known as the Alternative Nobel Prize). Her books include *Spiritual Midwifery, Ina May's Guide to Childbirth, Ina May's Guide to Breastfeeding, and Birth Matters: A Midwife's Manifesta*.

To learn more about Ina May Gaskin, watch the Award Winning Documentary "Birth Story" (watchbirthstorymovie.com)

ROBIN "IBU ROBIN" LIM (1956-present)

Lim is the founder of a free prenatal care and birth service center in Bali, Indonesia, called Yayasan Bumi Sehat (Healthy Mother Earth Foundation), and two others in Aceh, Indonesia and Tacloban, Philippines. Combined, the three clinics have facilitated the births of more than 5,000 babies. Robin and her team are working to combat Indonesia's high maternal and infant mortality rates. CNN awarded her "Hero of the Year" in 2011. Lim is a mother of eight children, and author of many books related to infant and maternal health, including: *Placenta: The Forgotten Chakra, The Ecology of Gentle Birth* and *After the Baby's Birth*. She stresses the importance of gentle birth as having an enormous effect on society.

SHEILA KITZINGER (1929–2015)

The "high priestess of natural childbirth" worked to change attitudes about childbirth, advocating that it should not be reduced to a pathological event, and waging a crusade against its medicalization. She believed birth should be seen and experienced as a highly potent, exhilarating, sensual event, and that problems in childbirth can be reduced through education. She promoted body awareness, relaxation techniques, and breathing patterns, and advocated the acceptance of labor pain, seeing it as a side effect of a task willingly undertaken. In 1962, Kitzinger came to prominence with the release of her book *The Experience of Childbirth*, addressing women's needs and choices as paramount. Until then, enemas, shaving, and episiotomies had been routine and regarded as essential, but as a result of her book, they were being questioned. Kitzinger wrote more than 30 books, translated into many languages, on birth, sexuality, breastfeeding, childcare, and motherhood. Her book *Pregnancy and Childbirth* has sold over a million copies.

AGNES GEREB (1952-present)

Agnes is a gynecologist, midwife, psychologist, and well-known homebirth attendant in Hungary (over 3,500 births). In 1977 she began smuggling fathers into labor rooms without permission, and as punishment banned from practicing for six months. Years later, the head of the clinic declared proudly that his institute was first to allow fathers into the labor room. Hungary is a country that has relentlessly pushed to criminalize homebirths and make hospital deliveries compulsory. There are just 15 homebirth midwives in Hungary; five of them currently face lengthy prison sentences. Geréb was charged with manslaughter when a baby died after a difficult labor, her license revoked for three years, and she became imprisoned on various charges. Gereb's story sparked international outrage. A heroine to women across Hungary, she dedicated 30 years to defending the right of mothers to choose their birthing experience. There is a film that includes her called *Freedom for Birth*.

MIDWIFE MEMOIRS
- Baby Catcher
- A Midwives Tale:
  The Life of Martha Ballard
- Call the Midwife
- Midwife: A Journey
- Labor of Love
- Arms Wide Open

INTERVIEW WITH A MIDWIFE

I interviewed a Certified Professional Midwife named Adrienne Leeds who began to study birth in 1999, and has attended births as a doula and midwife assistant since 2001. She embraces a holistic, flexible, mother-centered approach.

How and why did you become a midwife?

There was a time in my life when everyone around me told me I should become a midwife, or introduced me as a future midwife, or said that I had midwife energy. I thought they were all nuts, but then I decided to look into it a little more. It was a time in my life when lots of things were changing. I was embracing living green and gardening and composting. I lived next door to a midwife and her family. I started borrowing her books and asking her questions, and seeing her prepare and coming home tired and the impact it had on her family. She was the one who introduced me as a future midwife. Then I just started studying. I found a midwife to mentor me and became more and more interested in births. When I moved to South Carolina, I began attending births as a doula and as a birth assistant.

Can you tell me about your training?

Midwifery is a lineage passed from one woman to another. I did a course with a midwife in Colorado and then an additional course through the association of Texas midwives. There are different pathways to midwifery. When Ina Mae Gaskin was starting, that generation of women created a resurgence of midwifery in the US. They were self-educated by and large by mentors, but mostly they recreated modern day midwifery.

Only 8 percent of births are attended primarily by midwives in the United States. Where do you think midwifery is going?

I have seen an expansion of midwifery with more and more midwives becoming credentialed. South Carolina has more than doubled the number of licensed midwives in the past 15 years. Some believe that in the future, there will be fewer obstetricians, and midwives will be poised to fill the gap. Home births and out-of-hospital births are increasing as well. Two percent of the births in the United States are out-of-hospital, and the number increases every year.

What is the role of a midwife?

To be the wife's partner in the birthing process. It's not a hierarchical model; it's a partnership model. The midwife is there to provide information, physical and emotional support, and help the mother to find the information to make informed decisions about the care of her body and her baby. Midwifery is incredibly rewarding and challenging. In terms of the actual work, it is a beautiful intimate dance. I come into people's lives, get to know them in a very specific way, and get to be present for this amazing miracle as they either become a family or enlarge their family. Then gradually, we release our hands and go about our ways. And then we do it again and again with others. I feel like it challenges me to be a better person, too. It challenges me to grow all the time.

Do you feel like there is going to be a turn around or a birthing revolution, where birth isn't filled with as much fear and intervention as there is in our society today?

I feel like there are those who are choosing to birth naturally and unhindered, and there are those who are making fear-based choices. The realization of the rising C-section rate needing to be stopped gives me a lot of hope. I think some positive trends are happening about birth.

How does one find a midwife?

Information about midwives can be found on several different web sites: MANA, the Midwife Alliance of North America, is a great one and has lots of information and links to finding midwives. On the state level, one can search for state chapters of certified nurse-midwifery and certified professional midwifery organizations. Maternity Wise and Childbirth Connection are two great resources that talk about choices in childbirth.

What are some obstacles to practicing midwifery?

A lot of people don't know that there are licensed midwives who are licensed by the state (and are not registered nurses) going into people's homes privately and helping them birth their babies in a professional manner. I feel like perhaps they think we are in the woods with chickens and bloody sacrifices. They don't realize the training that we have to go through, about the prenatal care schedule, or that what we do at a prenatal visit is identical as to what an obstetrician would do. Midwives are indeed the guardians of a healthy pregnancy and normal birth. So in a sense, our skills in out-of-hospital birth settings are more considerable because we are trained in physiological birth. We see what's normal; we know what's normal. We can reassure people that, yes, this is indeed typical of what you are going through. I think there is a lot of fear around childbirth that is accepted, and someone who trains in a fear-based environment brings their fear to the table.

Those who train in a non-fear-based environment bring confidence in the woman and faith in themselves. Ina May delivered 180 babies before a C-section was necessary. She thought to herself, "Wow, this works!" She had experienced it. They told her with her first child that they needed to use forceps, and she felt it was unnecessary. So just that feeling that it can happen another way is perhaps what brought her to that moment in life where she became a midwife. I feel like my job is a guardian of holding the space, and keeping the space for normal birth means being able to open. Being somebody that people can be open around and have the oxytocin flow so that the baby can come forth in an environment of love.

Can you share some of the processes with the mother?

I have an initial consultation and interview with the woman. I encourage her and her partner to meet as many midwives as they like who are working in our communities so that they can find the right personality match. If we agree to start care together, we meet once a month until the third trimester and then every two weeks until 36 weeks, and then weekly. Some people have offices. I do my visits in the client's home, and I love getting to know people in that way. It's intimate, and I'm at ease in their space, and they are comfortable with me being there. When it's time for the birth, I usually look for a call or text that things are happening. We decide when I will come over when there is active labor, which happens night or day, as I am on call 24/7. Once there, I monitor the baby and the mother.

Are midwives only for home births?

Midwives work with women in hospitals, birthing centers, and at home. It depends on the state you are in and what your training is. In South Carolina, some nurse-midwives primarily work in hospitals and birthing center settings. In some states, nurse midwives also attend home births. Licensed midwives or direct-entry midwives, who are now becoming certified professionals, often work in an out-of-hospital setting, as they don't have hospital privileges. In the United Kingdom, when a woman finds out she is pregnant, she is assigned a midwife, and then the midwives have a very symbiotic relationship with the doctors and the hospitals. So there isn't as big of a gap as it seems there is here in the United States. Midwives work with low-risk women, and a mother only sees a specialist if she is in a high-risk category. In that sense, the midwives can excel in their area of expertise—low-risk births—and the specialist can excel in their area of expertise—high-risk scenarios such as surgery and surgical births. It is a win-win for everybody. It serves their population very well.

Can you speak a bit about oxytocin?

Oxytocin is a hormone that the body secretes from the pituitary gland when one is feeling love. It is secreted during sex, during menstruation, during childbirth, and during breastfeeding. Besides cultivating the feeling of love and bonding, it helps the uterus contract to expel the baby. So when oxytocin is high, adrenaline and fear hormones are low, and there is a nice warm fuzzy feeling in the room, and it helps the baby come. There is a French obstetrician named Michel Odant who speaks all over the world about oxytocin as the hormone of love. A lot of books suggest to kiss your partner while you are in labor and be intimate so that hormone can flow even stronger. The same hormones that help the baby come into being are the same hormones that can help the baby come out. Oxytocin is in a synthetic form called Pitocin that is very useful to help somebody stop bleeding. It can be a life-saving medication. It is not analogous to the oxytocin that comes from our bodies, as it doesn't cross the blood-brain barrier, so it doesn't create those same warm and fuzzy love feelings. Frequently, in a medical setting, there is less free-flowing innate oxytocin because it is either being used externally or because the environment is not conducive to it.

What are the primary positions that are used to give birth?
I facilitate a lot of water births. Women find birthing in a pool very comfortable—over 90% of my clients give birth in water. The woman can assume any position, and buoyancy helps when there is a big baby belly. People squat, they get on their hands and knees, sometimes they sit back and hold their legs out. I encourage people to find whatever position feels right for them. I am not usually too directive about it unless there is a need to be.

In hospitals, mothers are told they cannot eat or drink during labor, whereas midwives support the intake of small snacks and fluids to keep their energy up, so the mothers do not get too tired. Can you speak on this?
This is not evidenced-based but practiced in a hospital setting that women have orders on their chart to be NPO ("nil per os," or "nothing by mouth"). Sometimes ice chips, popsicles, or clear liquids are offered. The reasoning behind this, is that should there be a need for emergency surgery, you would have to undergo general anesthesia, and there is a small chance you would vomit and then aspirate the contents into the lungs and have a catastrophic event. So for that reason, they restrict feeding and fluids in women by mouth. Often mothers are given an IV for hydration while they are laboring in a hospital setting. But if you or I had just eaten lunch or dinner, were in

a car accident and needed surgery, no one would think twice about giving us the anesthesia and surgery needed in order to save our life. So it is a bit of a double standard.

One third of all births in the U.S. are now cesarean births and often scheduled before it is medically necessary. What are your thoughts on this?

I think the steps that the United States has taken to reduce the Cesarean rate are positive. There was a big campaign by the March of Dimes touting no inductions that aren't medically necessary before 39 weeks. I hear there is a new campaign to not induce until at least 40 weeks. So, they are trying to make sure that women and babies are ready for birth. New studies are coming to light all the time that the baby initiates the labor, which means waiting until the baby is fully developed. It's like how the tomato on the vine tastes best when it is ripe—let the baby ripen until it's ready and initiates the birthing process.

What is the role between the obstetrician and the midwife?

In South Carolina, all expecting mothers are required to have at least two visits with a consulting obstetrician or nurse-midwife. This facilitates the development of a relationship with the specialist and meets the checks and balances in terms of baby and mother being healthy and low risk and appropriate to having birth in an out-of-hospital setting. I am grateful to have a consulting OB that I can call and ask questions of and discuss some gray areas that come up, such as, for example, hypertension. If I see something unusual in a prenatal visit, I can share my plan, get her thoughts, and decide whether the mother is still eligible to continue with midwifery care. On a national level, the American Congress of Obstetricians and Gynecologists has come out against out-of-hospital births, specifically home births. They are supportive of birth center births and have acknowledged certified professional midwives as professionals who may work in a birth center setting, which is unprecedented. However, they have made a statement against home births that brings a lot of fear about it. One thing that would help is midwives becoming more integrated into the hospital setting. Then we could, for example, transport in clients who are at risk and be greeted as competent professionals instead of, "Who are you, where are you from, and why on Earth are you attempting birth out of hospital?" There is still a lot of education needed. There are a few shining stars in the medical field that are changing things and saying that we are here to support women who are birthing in all settings.

Can you speak about gentle birth?

Think of a new soul arriving on this planet for the very first time. They can hear their parents' voices and are surrounded by love. If they can go through their transition in an unhurried way, that feels right to their rhythm, so they can take in all the new sensations such as gravity, feeling the air in their lungs, the air around them, sounds, feelings, the skin of their mother, tastes, smells and everything they are being exposed to for the first time, releasing their cord and placenta when the time is right, that is gentleness. That big transition is extraordinary. To come into this world gently sows the seeds for non-violence throughout their lives.

What do you want to say to women out there who are pregnant or thinking of becoming pregnant?

Trust yourselves. Trust your intuition. Find that space so that you can hear your voice, and find people around you who will support you in speaking your voice.

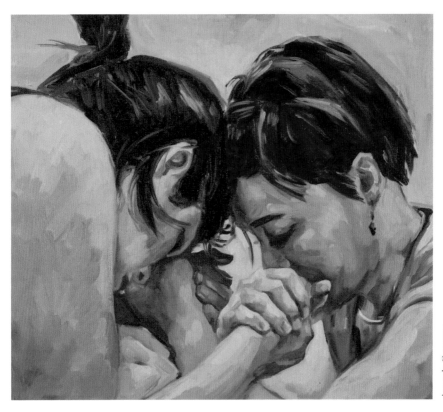

Amanda Greavette

CHAPTER 3: DOULAS

"...Respecting the woman as an important and valuable human being and making certain that the woman's experience while giving birth is fulfilling and empowering is not just a nice extra, it is absolutely essential as it makes the woman strong and therefore makes society strong."
- MARSDEN WAGNER

"The whole point of woman-centered birth is the knowledge that a woman is the birth power source. She may need, and deserve, help, but in essence, she always had, currently has, and will have the power."
- HEATHER MCCUE

BEING A DOULA HAS been another gift for my ever-expanding awareness of the spirit. I can't recall when I found out what a doula was, but now I am one! The first birth I attended was a mother's second baby, at the local birth center, with her husband, midwife, and myself. She was in the tub, and as I knelt in front of her, I remember her saying, "Help me," as she got closer to the birth. So I did. Doula-ing is a service of being intuitive, attentive, and positive, with a fierce conviction of a mother's (and baby's) inner wisdom and power. Doulas have a role that lends to advocating for a mother's rights, options, and decisions. If the care providers are not treating a woman with dignity or honoring her wishes, the doula is a third party witness, who can assist in shifting the energy and often the outcome. Doulas are with the mother the entire labor and birthing process. The longest for me to date has been 23 hours straight in a hospital. The nurses and doctor changed shifts three times, and I was there for the entirety. Some nurses and doctors are welcoming and appreciative of doulas, and others not.

WHAT IS A DOULA?

A doula is a professional trained in childbirth who provides emotional, physical, and informational support to the mother who is expecting, is experiencing labor, or has recently given birth. The doula's purpose is to help women have a safe, memorable, and empowering birthing experience.

A labor and birth doula will help you understand the birthing sensations and help you decide when to call your midwife or head to the hospital. They will help you set up the birth pool, get comfortable, remind you to breathe, squeeze your hips, massage your back, help clean up postpartum, and more.

WHAT DOULAS DO

Doulas usually offer a consultation with the mother and partner, to answers questions, ensure it is a good fit, and briefly discuss fees and services. The meeting is about 30 minutes to an hour. If hired, the doula may offer two prenatal visits, during which she and the parents will get to know one another, review birth wishes, explore labor coping techniques, discuss reading material and postpartum care, etc. She is then available for support until 38 weeks, and on-call 24/7 up to and through the birth.

Doulas provide information and resources on labor and childbirth and give mother and partner physical, emotional, and spiritual support during active labor and delivery. They usually secure a back-up doula that is on call in case they cannot attend or will be late to the labor for some reason. Most doulas stay after the birth for an hour or two helping out and will make one or more postpartum visits to check on the mother and review the birth details.

WHAT DOULAS DO NOT DO

Doulas do not perform clinical tasks such as cervical exams, or anything pertaining to the medical side of labor and birth. It is the mother's time to enforce her wishes. The doula is there to help the mother and partner navigate through it all, and ensure she is informed, respected, treated well, and listened to by caregivers, so that her choices, wishes, and vision are an integral part of the experience. The doula will offer suggestions and advice, but the mother is the ultimate decision-maker.

DOULA FEES

Birth doula fees range anywhere from $400–$2,000, with an average of $1,200. Postpartum doulas usually charge by the hour, around $35. The fee can depend on the city, as well as different packages and offerings.

Doulas and midwives stay in town for 2 weeks before and after the guess date, scheduling around the birth. If you interview with a doula or midwife, but decide not to hire her, as a courtesy let her know as soon as you can with a quick text, email, or phone call.

INTERVIEW WITH A DOULA

The interview below is with Maria Petrie, a DONA (Doulas of North America) trained birth doula. She is also trained in homeopathy for childbirth, the Bradley Method, and Hypnobabies, and is in process of becoming a nurse-midwife.

What does the word "doula" mean?
It is a Greek word that means "woman servant." It came into place in the United States in the late 1970s. They were first using doulas in South America.

How did you become a doula?
Most women who become doulas find the route of becoming a doula through birthing their child. They have a very empowering birth experience, and they want to help other women have a great experience as well. Or sometimes maybe they didn't have an ideal experience and want to help educate other women to have a better experience. I am a bit more unique because I don't have children yet. I was working in a different career full time and considering changing careers entirely to one in women's health in a more clinical role. Then I was having lunch with a friend who had just come from the birth of her sister, and her sister had a doula. It was the first time that I had ever heard the word, and she explained what this woman did during the birth. I was living in Washington, DC at that time and was fortunate to find out there was a training only three weeks later. In March of 2012, I completed the training with DONA, the oldest training organization. I attended my first birth three months later and have since been to almost 50 births. I have

accompanied many families in all kinds of settings: hospitals, birth centers, and homes.

There are birth doulas and postpartum doulas, correct?

That's right. Many doulas do both kinds of work. I am a birth doula only. A birth doula has more training and specializes in attending the labor and delivery, while a postpartum doula is skilled in newborn care, and comes in on an hourly basis, or custom-fits a plan to meet whatever the family's needs are.

How much before the actual birth of the baby are you with the family? What is the process?

It varies on when the family might reach out to me. Ideally, I like to meet a family around 28 to 30 weeks of pregnancy. Most birth doulas include two prenatal appointments. Those are about two hours each in the family's home where we spend some time getting to know each other.

We might talk about any childbirth education classes they have taken. It is important that both the mother and father understand the physiology of birth. Also, I learn what their goals are in terms of the birth. Do they plan a medicated birth? Who do they want to be there? How do they envision each person's role? What things does the father do and what does the doula do? These are all things we go over during those visits.

In addition to the education that happens, it is an opportunity for us to get together so we can be an effective team on the day of delivery. Generally, I talk to my clients weekly and then daily depending on how things are going. If the mom is approaching her date and feeling anxious, we might communicate more often. Whenever she feels like things are kicking off, I join the family as soon as they are ready for support. Sometimes it is very early on in labor, especially for first-time parents, or it could be when things are actively moving on.

The critical service that doulas provide is continuous support. I think many new families are surprised to find how often they are left alone. In your place of birth, your clinical providers generally have other patients and responsibilities, and they might need to leave the room even for just a little while. Especially for first-time parents, this can be disconcerting. So having someone in the room with you reassuring you that everything is normal is generally comforting. Especially for dads so there is not so much pressure on them to be the only coach. I stay with the family throughout the entire labor and delivery and about an hour or two after. I get everyone settled; we work on first latch to get breastfeeding initiated, then I leave everyone to rest. I usually come back around day three to check on the mom, see how breastfeeding is going, and talk about postpartum healing.

Do you work in different environments: hospitals, birthing centers and home births?
I do. Most doulas attend births in all settings. The priority is attending the woman in the birth setting where she feels comfortable.

What is the training like for a doula?
There are several different training organizations. Generally speaking, there are a few days of classroom training, a body of reading, a written test, and an experiential component. In the first three births that you work with, the doctor or midwife and the mother fill out forms that you turn into your training organization, which speaks about your performance as a doula.

What is your relationship with midwives?
We frequently work together with midwives. The main distinction between a midwife and a doula is that a midwife has a clinical role. Thus, the midwife is primarily responsible for the safety of mother and baby. In a home birth setting, the midwife can also focus on providing physical and emotional support. However, in a hospital or birth center, the midwife might have other mothers to attend to, so the doula can be there to support the mother. Midwives and doulas have very different, but complementary roles.

What are some of the things that you recommend to mothers for postpartum care?
I feel that there is a lot of pressure in our culture to return to "normal life" very quickly. This pressure interferes with the necessity of a new mother's rest. Labor and delivery is an incredible physical feat. It is best in the postpartum period for the mother to rest, eat a lot of nutritious food, ask for

help, and have a plan for who will do things around the house, which she usually does, including care of the older children.

What about the expense of having a doula?
It is an expense that is worth prioritizing! The fee primarily covers the unpredictability of being on call. We are on-call and available to the mother 24/7 for questions and concerns for up to five weeks, in addition to being ready to join them for the birth within an hour's notice and remaining with them through the entire labor, whether short or long. The prenatal education component and connecting the family with resources available to them in town, such as postpartum support or lactation consultants is valuable.

Have you ever considered being a postpartum doula?
I enjoy the birth doula role and the prenatal education component of working with parents before their birth and making the birth experience good for everyone. When it comes to newborn care, my role as a doula is to connect the family with the resources available to them in town, such as postpartum support or lactation consultants.

One of the many ways one can help prevent postpartum depression is to ingest the placenta. That is becoming more popular, and there are different techniques available. Can you speak on this subject?
In addition to the benefits of the placenta, what we highlighted earlier about rest and proper nutrition for the mom is vital for a healthy and successful postpartum period. If you're interested in encapsulating your placenta, it provides a restoration of iron and natural hormones that moms find offer an incredible balance in the postpartum period. It's not necessary to have experienced postpartum depression or be fearful that you might. It can be more preventive and may help curb a potential problem or make you feel excellent if you were already going to feel normal. It is pretty much all benefit and no risk. If you feel well supported and have a good labor and birth experience, that in and of itself can help prevent postpartum depression.

Are doulas usually full time or part time doulas?

I have a full-time job and am a part-time doula, which limits the number of clients I can serve each month. Some doulas are full-time doulas. There are all different models out there.

How many mothers a month does a full-time doula serve?

I would say about five per month.

If the mom has older children, are they ever present at the birth of the new baby?

On occasion. It depends upon the place of birth. Homebirth is very friendly to that. It also depends on the age of the child. At the hospital, the children usually come afterward. In the birth center, it is somewhere in between the two.

Can you take us through a birth scenario, giving an example of what occurs on your end?

It varies widely. Generally speaking, I will provide phone support early on. Mom might call and say she thinks things might be starting. I will advise her to take a warm bath, relax, and keep me informed. Then I'll get a text from the partner, who will say things are starting to progress and ask for me to come over. So I get there, and I am comfortable there. I already know the family. I walk in and go into the space where the mom is and see the energy in the room. Is she laughing? Do things seem like they are pretty early on? How much attention is each of the pressure waves requiring? If we need to speed things up, we might go outside for a walk, or I might suggest a change of position. We revisit that every hour or so until the body takes over. Generally, moms will move into a position that feels good. At that point, if they are having a hospital birth, we may go to hospital. Or if there is a midwife, she shows up or is already there.

Anything else you wish to add?

Doulas are not just for moms planning a non-medicated birth. Just like we serve women in all settings, we work with all sets of births plans. If you are planning a medicated birth or a Cesarean, a doula can still be an asset to you both during the labor and birth and especially during your postpartum period.

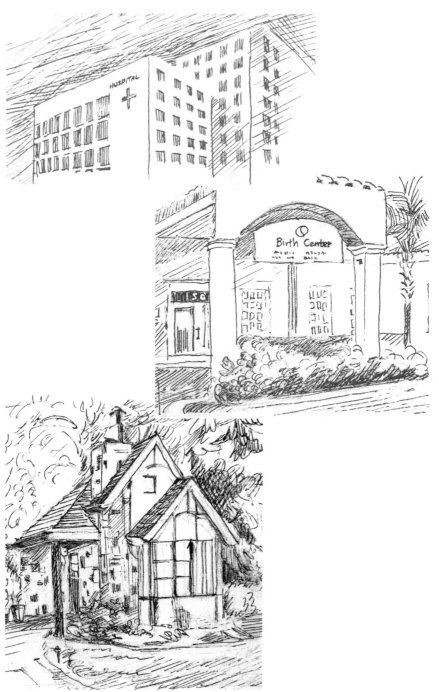

CHAPTER 4:
BIRTHING LOCATIONS

"Giving birth should be your greatest achievement, not your greatest fear."
- JANE WEIDEMAN

"Whenever and however you give birth, your experience will impact your emotions, your mind, your body, and your spirit for the rest of your life."
- INA MAY GASKIN,
Midwife

"Women don't really need to be taught how to birth. They simply need to learn about birth. They come to understand that when the mind is free of stress and fear that cause the body to respond with pain, nature is free to process birth in the same well-designed manner that it does for all other normal physiological functions."
- MARIE MONGAN

IN LABOR, A WOMAN is navigating through the sensations, uncertainty, and sensitivity to her surroundings. The words she hears spoken to her and around her, the tones of voice, any touch to her body she feels, are all heightened in the hours of labor. Whoever is with her during these hours will play a role in the outcome of her birthing experience. No mother wants to feel fear, pressure, disrespect, doubt, worry, or disregard when working to birth her baby. A mother will play the birth over in her head time and again. The place she chooses should be based on where she is most comfortable, and anyone in that environment should make sure she is comfortable and treated like a goddess.

Did you know that the United States spends more money on pregnancy and childbirth technology than any other country on this planet? Yet 33% of the childbirths in the U.S. are Cesarean sections. The U.S. is the only country on Earth with a rising maternal mortality rate, despite the high price of health-care, and has the 4th highest infant maternal mortality rate (after Mexico, Chile, and Turkey) compared with 34 other developed countries, according to the Organization for Economic Co-operation and Development. Paradoxically, many women in the United States don't have insurance or the finances to pay for Obstetrics/Gynecological care, hospital bills, prenatal vitamins, etc.

BIRTHING OPTIONS

A woman's birthing experience can and should be as unique and personal as she wants it to be. She can choose to be in the bathtub or shower during labor, in a birthing pool, at a hospital, at home, or a birthing center. She can choose to touch the baby's head as he or she emerges and even reach down and bring them out. A woman can opt to keep her baby with her instead of being taken to be weighed, to not cut the umbilical cord, to turn off bright lights, to have minimal medical staff in the room, to leave baby unwashed, etc.

The most important thing to remember: it is the woman who brings the baby through her body. She births the baby into the world, and the doctor, midwife, or partner, is the one who catches the baby. To have the baby "delivered" insinuates that the mother is the recipient of the action rather than the agent. The mother is doing the labor, the work, and has the innate wisdom and ability to birth her child. Suppressing this intrinsic wisdom, the woman's intuition, or doubting the capability of a mother to birth is a great disservice to society. The potent, cosmic, and magical event of birth happens every 2.5 seconds, about 130 million times a year around the world. Our power as women to form another life within our bodies is too vast to comprehend. Birthing new life is a sacred event. The mother is not sick or a patient; she is bringing forth a soul and contributing to the continuation of humanity.

HERSTORY OF BIRTH LOCATIONS

Currently, in the US, 99% of babies are born in hospitals. Delivering at home or independent birthing centers is not yet close to being considered mainstream. But it hasn't always been this way.

৵

In 1900: About 95% of births took place at home. After 1900, more women were attracted to hospitals because hospitals could offer medicated birth not available in homebirths.

1927: 85% of births took place at home.

1933: The White House Conference on Child Health and Protection issued a report stating that maternal mortality had not declined between 1915 and 1930, despite the increase in hospital births, introduction of prenatal care and wider use of techniques to minimize contamination. During this time, the number of infant deaths from birth injuries increased by about 50% because women received little or no prenatal care, or received excessive interventions that were incorrectly performed.

1935: 37% percent of births occurred in hospitals.

	Home Birth	Birthing Center	Hospital
Cost*	$2500–$4500	$3000–$8000	$3,296–$37,227

*with and without insurance

1938: By this time, doctors used "twilight sleep" in all births. Twilight sleep is a condition induced by an injection of morphine and scopolamine, which produces a semi-narcotic state, and an experience of childbirth without the pain, memory of pain, or the birth.

1939: 50% of all women and 75% of all urban women delivered in hospitals.

1950: 88% of births occurred in hospitals.

1960: 97% of births occurred in hospitals.

2017: 99% of births occur in hospitals.

HOSPITAL

Many hospitals have within them a Labor and Delivery unit. Every hospital is different, with some being more cooperative with the mother's wishes than others. Most women are placed in a bed on their backs and offered drugs. While some women successfully deliver this way, it is not the only birthing position. But sometimes, it is presented to the mother as the only option. Many OBGYNs are not accustomed to women birthing any other way and thereby will ask the mother to accommodate this norm by being on the bed. If the mother chooses an epidural, it will limit her birthing positions, and most likely confine her to delivering her baby in bed. There's no way to squat, kneel, or sit up if you can't feel your legs.

INTRAVENOUS FLUIDS

One of the first things presented at the hospital is an IV. Intravenous therapy is used to place fluids directly in the mother's veins, and it is standard procedure for doctors to insert an IV even in a low-risk delivery, because if there is an emergency, the IV will already be set to administer medication. However, an IV can easily be inserted if necessary in the case of an emergency. So long as the mother is hydrated, and continues to drink, she will receive fluids in this way. IV bags are attached to a pole on wheels that you have to drag around with you, limiting movement. If the mother declines an IV, she is usually urged to receive a Heparin lock, which is an intravenous catheter threaded into a peripheral vein, flushed with saline, and capped off. This way she is not hooked up to an IV pole, but there is now easy access for injecting something later. The mother may be told that it is "standard policy" or "routine," but it is not policy, and she can decline the Hep-lock, as well as any other "standard policies." Signing consent forms on the way into the hospital does not mean she is giving "informed consent." The mother can say no to any of these routine procedures.

ELECTRICAL FETAL MONITORING

Two wide stretchy bands holding electronic disks called transducers will be wrapped around the mother's back and placed against her abdomen. One monitors the baby's heartbeat and the other tracks contractions. This is called continuous electrical fetal monitoring (EFM). It is used to let the nurses and doctor know the heart accelerations and decelerations, whether the baby is stressed in any way, and when contractions are coming and going. The constant monitoring itself, though, has not been shown to increase positive health results for the babies and can increase the chances of a C-section, forceps, and vacuum delivery. Studies have shown that mothers monitored intermittently throughout labor birthed babies as successfully and healthy as women who were constantly monitored. False-positive electronic fetal monitoring readings—which indicate a problem when the baby is actually fine—do occur.

Some researchers believe that the majority of decelerations, or rapid falls in fetal heart rate, are normal and not dangerous. A healthy fetus could be adapting to brief but repeated periods of low oxygen during contractions by triggering the peripheral chemoreflex. Chemoreflexes are an essential mechanism for the regulation of both breathing and autonomic cardiovascular function. This notion explains why many babies are born healthy despite repeated brief decelerations during labor. What qualifies as normal fetal heart rate patterns during labor is broader than previously thought.

Many moms-to-be find EFM uncomfortable and limiting. It can be more challenging to cope with contractions with transducers strapped to the belly. The sensors slide down often, require frequent adjustments by nurses, and can cause inaccurate readings on the monitors, which then creates stress. Beltless, wireless monitors (like the Novii) are a new invention and becoming popular in hospitals, with sticker patches placed on the belly that transmit data via Bluetooth technology. The safety, security, and viability of such technology has yet to be tested or established. The doctor will likely require constant fetal monitoring during labor if the mother has anemia, low amniotic fluid, a history of heart disease, diabetes, hyperthyroidism, obesity, preeclampsia, is carrying multiples, or goes into labor before 37 weeks or after 42 weeks. Also, if there is meconium stain, the baby is in a breech position (feet or buttocks first), or the mother is "high risk." The mother can call the hospital and have them read aloud their policy for constant fetal monitoring and what constitutes high risk, or have it shown in writing.

A mom can request intermittent fetal monitoring or hands-on listening if she has had a low-risk pregnancy and no complications in labor. Periodic fetal monitoring is performed at intervals, usually with transducers or a handheld

Doppler device. Hands-on listening is when the baby's heartbeat is checked with a Doppler or fetoscope for at least 60 seconds every 15–30 minutes or so during the active phase of the first stage of labor, and at least 5–15 minutes during the pushing phase of the second stage of labor (ACNM 2015).

Fetal monitors detect fetal heart rate externally by using an ultrasound transducer to transmit and receive ultrasonic waves. An ultrasonic wave is defined as an "inaudible sound with high frequency for human" which generally exceeds 20 kilohertz, and is not intended to be heard. Infants have particularly acute hearing, and the speed of sound in longitudinal waves is over four times higher in water than air. The baby is in water; therefore, it may be stressful for them, and it is vital to consider the baby's experience in labor. (See Ultrasound Chapter for more on this topic).

FACTORS OF ENVIRONMENT

The hospital experience includes abundant stimulation, with anesthesiologists coming in to offer drugs, nurses constantly checking on you and the monitors, the doctor coming in to do cervical exams, etc. The lighting in the hospital room will be bright, though you can have the lights turned down or off (you could even bring a lamp), and close the curtain if there is a window. The small room might contain the obstetrician, multiple registered nurses, neonatologists, anesthesiologists, medical students, and other health care professionals. Interestingly, the mother is given a limit as to how many support people she is "allowed" to have. Usually, the partner is not allowed to accompany the mother to the operating room in the case of a C-section and is the only one who can be present in the room for the procedure.

Women are not encouraged to eat or drink in the hospital setting. The old school of thought was that food in the digestive system could cause the mother to aspirate. Also, if she needs emergency anesthesia, doctors are afraid of her choking on the food. In truth, even if she does require anesthesia, it's not likely she will have issues with aspiration.

Most hospitals and doctors these days are not supportive of vaginal breech deliveries, even though the baby can rotate in labor up until the last minute from breech to head first. Many hospitals have a ban that prohibits women from attempting a vaginal birth after Cesarean.

Some hospitals have squat bars, birthing balls, a standard tub, shower, and rocking chairs. It is now becoming popular to add birthing suites that provide more of a home-like setting.

With a hospital birth, the nurses will attempt to take the baby from the mother at various times for specific procedures (weighing, footprints, etc.) and likely to a different room for his or her first checkup. The mother can refuse. Baby can stay with the mother for as long as she likes. These things can happen with the mother holding the baby, or right next to her bed while she still is holding/touching the child.

If a mother plans to birth in a hospital, she must know their policies beforehand (ask for a printout). She must not be afraid to challenge them and voice her wants and needs (repeatedly if need be). Having a support team there will help make sure she is getting what she wants, and not getting what she doesn't want, as much as is possible.

HOSPITAL CHARGES

It may surprise you how much the bill can vary. A recent University of California, San Francisco study found that the cost of uncomplicated vaginal births in California varied between hospitals by as much as $34,000, ranging from $3,296 to $37,227 for on-site hospital costs.

On average, the cost of having a baby in the U.S. without complications is $10,808 per stay, according to the most recent survey data from the International Federation of Health Plans (April 2018). Add in prenatal, delivery-related and postpartum health-care, and you are looking at an $18,383 tab. "Childbirth is one of the most expensive payouts for insurance companies, and more than 300,000 American women give birth every month," says Sarah O'Leary of Exhale Healthcare Advocates, a national consumer health-care advocacy group. Since insurance companies make money by taking in more than they pay out, their customers often have to shoulder some—or a lot—of the financial burden.

The U.S. is by far the most expensive place in the world to give birth or receive medical treatment, because there are no publicly financed health services like most developed countries have. Since prices are higher, patients receive more services, according to Prof. Gerard Anderson of the Johns Hopkins Center for Hospital Finance and Management. "If you can make more money as a doctor by ordering more tests, you are going to order them. Therefore, patients end up getting more tests," he says. It also increases revenue for the hospitals. Costs of birthing in a hospital may include but are not limited to: ultrasounds, episiotomy, epidural, circumcision, and overnight stay.

BIRTH CENTER

The American Association of Birth Centers defines a birth center as a home-like setting where care providers, usually midwives, provide family-centered care to healthy pregnant women. Besides being a place for birth, they typically offer well-woman exams, preconception counseling, prenatal care, lactation education/classes/consulting, childbirth education, women's health information, breastfeeding, and infant massage classes. Most birth centers are located separately from hospitals, while a few are physically inside hospital buildings, but separate from the Labor and Delivery unit.

In birth centers, midwives and staff provide continuous, supportive care, and interventions like fetal monitors and IV fluids are used only when medically necessary. Women are encouraged to eat if they are hungry, move about and spend time in a tub as they wish, and birth in whatever positions they find most comfortable. Birth centers recognize that the mother knows what her body needs to give birth. The midwives and staff attend to her needs, while diligently watching for signs that are outside the realm of wellness. In the U.S., 0.3% of births take place in birth centers.

Procedures that are standard or at least common in a hospital setting (such as continuous fetal monitoring, IV, induction) aren't routine at a birth center. Birth centers do not offer epidurals but do have options such as hydrotherapy, breathing exercises, massage, acupuncture, and sometimes nitrous oxide gas. Pitocin is on hand for administration in case of postpartum hemorrhage. Birthing centers also have IVs, oxygen, and infant resuscitators on hand for use in case of a hospital transfer.

One study showed that 94% of women who entered labor at a birth center achieved a vaginal birth. In other words, the C-section rate was only 6%. Of the 15,574 women who planned to birth at the birth center at the start of labor: 84% birthed at the birth center and 16% were transferred to a nearby hospital in labor (due to extremely difficult labor/fatigue)—1% of those transferred for emergency reasons.

Most families leave the center four to eight hours after birth, compared to 24 to 48 hours at a hospital.

BIRTH CENTER CHARGES

The cost for prenatal care and birthing at a birth center is around $3000–$8000, varying according to where you live and the place you choose. Birthing centers handle only low-risk pregnancies. If the mother has hypertension, diabetes, gestational diabetes, is pregnant with multiples, or there are other issues that may cause complications, a birthing center is likely not an option. Birth centers also may have restriction on breech delivery.

HOME

Home sweet home. Many people in the United States view labor as a mine-field of disaster waiting to happen, so home birth is rare these days. But as you read earlier, that was how it was for millennia. Research supports that home birth is indeed safe. The mistrust of home births began in 1978 when the American College of Obstetricians and Gynecologists released a widely published report stating that births that did not happen in a hospital posed a two-to-five time greater risk to a baby's life. But their report was faulty, as the research included *all* out-of-hospital births, which included: unattended births, those en route to the hospital, mothers who were high risk, had no prenatal care, were preterm, and even miscarriages! So, planned attended homebirths involving healthy, full-term, low-risk mothers were lumped together with all of these!

Less than 1% of American women give birth at home. So for every 100 of your friends and family members who get pregnant and have a baby, 99 of them will birth in a hospital. It is legal in all 50 states for parents to have the baby where and with whom they desire, yet each state has different requirements as to whether or not it is legal for a midwife to assist a family in a homebirth.

LARGEST STUDY TO DATE

In the largest ever examination of planned home births in the U.S., it was found that among low-risk women, planned home births resulted in low rates of interventions, without increasing adverse outcomes for mothers and newborns. The study, titled "Outcomes of Care for 16,924 Planned Home Births in the United States: The Midwives Alliance of North America Statistics Project, 2004 to 2009," looked at nearly 17,000 women and their newborns. It found that for planned home births with a midwife in attendance:

- The rate of normal physiologic birth was over 93%
- The cesarean rate was 5.2%
- The rate of vacuum or forceps-assisted vaginal birth was 1.2%
- Less than 5% of mothers required oxytocin augmentation or epidural analgesia
- Only 1.5% of newborns had a low Apgar score (a measure of newborn health in the first five minutes following birth)
- 2.5% of newborns were admitted to the intensive care unit (NICU) at some point during the first six weeks following birth
- 87% of women with a previous cesarean (VBAC) delivered their newborns vaginally
- Of the 10.9% of women who transferred from home to hospital during labor, the majority changed locations for non-emergent reasons, such as a slow, non-progressing labor, or maternal exhaustion
- At six weeks postpartum, more than 97% of newborns were partially breastfed, and 86% were exclusively breastfed

*Study performed by Melissa Cheyney Ph.D., CPM, LDM, Marit Bovbjerg Ph.D., MS, Courtney, Everson MA, Wendy Gordon MPH, CPM, LM, Darcy Hannibal Ph.D., Saraswathi Vedam CNM, MSN, R.M. and first published January 30, 2014

"These rates of intervention are significantly lower than those seen in U.S. hospitals, without a simultaneous increase in adverse outcomes," said Dr. Melissa Cheyney, lead author on the study. The study, released in the Journal of Midwifery & Women's Health (JMWH), was conducted by researchers at Oregon State University, Bastyr University, the University of California Davis, and the University of British Columbia, and based on a voluntary dataset collected by the Midwives Alliance of North America. The MANA statistics registry contains high-quality data that uses the gold standard—the medical record—instead of birth certificate data, which research shows is unreliable for studying intended place of birth and newborn outcomes. "Our goal was to design a dataset that could help to reliably inform health care providers, policy makers, and families about the outcomes of midwifery care in all birth settings, and the characteristics of normal physiologic birth," said Geraldine Simkins, Executive Director, Midwives Alliance of North America. "Planned home births are only a small percentage of all births in the U.S., but the numbers are growing each year. Given these data, we hope providers in all settings can learn from what's working well at planned home births."

GOOD CANDIDATES FOR HOMEBIRTH:
(this should not be considered an exhaustive list):
- Pregnant with a single baby
- Healthy overall, eating a healthy prenatal diet, non-smoker
- Able to envision an active role in giving birth with minimal intervention, willing to cope with the work of labor (without drugs)
- Lives where midwives are available, are laboring within 30 minutes of a hospital and can cover expenses (as insurance is most often limited to hospital births)
- Baby is head down at term
- Between 37 and 42 weeks pregnant
- No serious medical conditions (heart disease, kidney disease, blood clotting disorders, type I diabetes, gestational diabetes managed with insulin, preeclampsia, or bleeding)
- No placenta previa at the beginning of labor
- No active genital herpes
- No thick meconium
- No prior C-section
- Spontaneous labor

HOMEBIRTH CHARGES
Around $2500–$4500, which includes prenatal care, attending labor and birth, and several postpartum visits.

WHAT DO MOTHERS SAY?
One study found that 91% of women who had had their last baby at home would prefer to have their next one at home. Among those who had had both a hospital birth and a homebirth, 76% preferred the home birth. Many people today consider home birth to be foolish, and others think it's brave. Here are some reasons one might choose a homebirth:
- Belief that home birth is safer than the hospital
- Desire to avoid unnecessary interventions
- Previous negative or traumatic hospital birth experience
- Control over birth decisions and choices
- Dislike of hospitals, doctors, or medically managed birth
- Desire for privacy and to avoid strangers
- Trust in childbirth as a normal, healthy process
- Lack of separation from baby, easier breastfeeding initiation
- Preference for midwives as caregivers
- Increased options such as delayed cord cutting or water birth
- Decreased risk of Cesarean operation
- Comfortable atmosphere
- Family involvement during the birth (children can be present)
- Reduced risk of infection
- History of precipitous labor where it is difficult to get to a hospital in time
- Infants born at home have more diverse bacteria in their guts and feces (microbiota) which positively affects their developing immunity and metabolism

The human microbiome consists of trillions of bacteria, fungi, and viruses that live on and in our bodies, many of which benefit our health and prevent chronic conditions such as obesity, diabetes, asthma, and gut inflammatory disorders. Microbes transmitted from mother to baby help prevent chronic disease.

"The reasons for the differences between infants born at home versus in hospitals are not known, but we speculate that common hospital interventions like early infant bathing and antibiotic eye prophylaxis or environmental factors—like the aseptic environment of the hospital—may be involved," says senior author Maria Gloria Dominguez-Bello, a professor of microbiome and health at Rutgers University. (Science Daily.com)

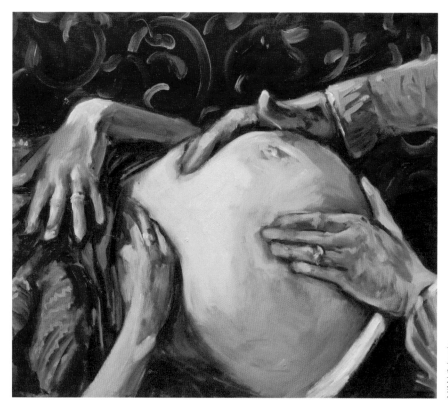

Nikki Scioscia

CHAPTER 5: QUESTIONS FOR CAREGIVERS

"Experiences have clearly shown that an approach which 'de-medicalizes' birth, restores dignity and humanity to the process of childbirth, and returns control to the mother is also the safest approach."

— MICHEL ODENT, MD

"If there is one thing you can do RIGHT NOW to ensure your best birth experience, it's this: Choose a care provider who is an EXPERT in the type of birth you are planning. If you're planning a safe, natural, unmedicated birth, you should hire someone who is an EXPERT at supporting natural birth. A doctor with a 30% C-section rate is not a natural birth expert. Neither is a doctor who does routine episiotomies, or doesn't understand how to catch a baby unless mom is lying on her back. A doctor who says, "Well, most of my clients do end up choosing an epidural, but if you want to go natural you can do that, I suppose..." is NOT an expert in unmedicated birth."

— LAURALYN CURTIS

SOME OF US ARE more inquisitive by nature. Curious about the who, what, when, and why (where is the where?) How will you find out? When it comes to choosing a caregiver, think of your birth like planning a huge event. You hire a venue, someone for the flower arrangements, the cake, the music, etc. This is way bigger than that. So if you put a lot of planning into a wedding, or birthday, or anniversary party, why wouldn't the birth of your child be given the utmost consideration as to who, what, when, where, and why? Asking questions is not being a nag or difficult. It is being responsible, informed, and empowered. Ask. If you get an answer that merits another question, ask again. An example:

Doctor: I don't want you going past 40 weeks.
Mother: Why?
Doctor: Because I don't like mothers to go past their due date.
Mother: But I am healthy, the baby is doing okay, right? So, why not wait?
Doctor: Because there are risks like the baby might be too big or they run out of amniotic fluid. It is best to go ahead and schedule a day for induction.
Mother: Why?

∽

If a health care provider becomes impatient or dismissive with your questions, then you have your answer already. If a potential health care provider makes you feel uneducated or fearful of the birth process, you can thank them, say goodbye, and find someone else.

QUESTIONS TO ASK AN OBGYN
- How many years have you been practicing?
- What is your philosophy about birth?
- What is your induction rate?
- What is the percentage of mothers who receive drugs (Pitocin, epidurals) in labor?
- Do you encourage drug-free births?
- What is your C-section rate?
- What are your opinions on declining continuous electronic fetal monitoring and/or IV fluids?
- How many cervical exams on average do you usually perform while a mother is in labor?
- Do you support vaginal breech birth?
- Do you require the gestational diabetes test? Is there an alternative to the Glucola drink?
- Do you test for GBS+? What is the course of treatment if a mom is positive?
- How often do mothers bring doulas to births with you?

- Do you practice delayed cord clamping and cutting? If so, how long do you usually wait?
- Do you practice immediate skin to skin for mother and child?
- Do you support a mother's desire to postpone weighing, footprints, bracelet, etc. for the baby until she is ready?
- I want to birth in any position that I feel. Are you supportive of this?
- Will you support my going to 42 weeks or even a few days past if all is well with baby and myself? What is the longest a mother has gone before they birthed with you as their OBGYN?
- Do you perform episiotomies? If so, how often?
- What about forceps usage?
- Do you support lotus birth?
- Do you support VBAC (if you are trying for one)

QUESTIONS TO ASK A MIDWIFE

- How many years have you been practicing?
- How many babies do you catch on average yearly?
- Where did you receive certification?
- Are you state licensed?
- How often will I have appointments scheduled?
- What happens during our appointments?
- Do you offer a payment plan and what do your fees include?
- Do you have/use a fetoscope?
- Do you require the use of dopplers?
- What lab work is needed?
- Do you require an ultrasound or vaginal exams?
- Do you require the gestational diabetes test? Is there an alternative to the Glucola drink?
- Do you test for GBS+? What is the course of treatment if a mom is positive?
- Do you offer home births? Water births?
- Do you do VBACs? What is your success rate?
- Do you support delayed cord clamping and cutting?
- Have you completed training in neonatal resuscitation?
- How do you handle situations when the baby is breech during labor?

- Do you have experience with postpartum hemorrhage, shoulder dystocia, breech baby or cord prolapse?
- How long after the guess date can a mother go in your care?
- At what point does a mother become too high risk for you to work with her?
- Which hospital(s) are you approved for working in case of an emergency?
- Which physicians are you affiliated with in case of transfer? Do you have personal relationships with them?
- What are some reasons that you would do a transfer?
- What percent of mothers end up with an epidural? With a Cesarean?
- Do you have children yourself? Did you use a midwife during your own births?

QUESTIONS TO ASK A DOULA

- What kind of training do you have?
- What is your philosophy about birth?
- How would you describe your doula style?
- Why did you become a doula?
- How do you most often support women in labor?
- How many births have you attended?
- What are your fees? What is included?
- Have you ever given birth, and, if so, what did you learn from your birth experience?
- Have you attended births at my birth location, and what was your experience there?
- Do you have any other mothers with due dates near mine?
- Do you have a backup doula? If so, may I meet her? How often is your backup doula used?
- Do you make any visits before the birth?
- Do you offer any postpartum care or follow up?
- May I email, text or call you with questions?
- Are you always on call once we decide to work together?
- Do you have experience with birth complications?
- Have you attended births that have ended up as a C-section?
- Have you attended home births?

- At what point in labor would you join me?
- Do you stay for the entire labor and childbirth, or do you have a time limit for long births?
- How do you work with the partner?
- How do you work with a midwife or doctor?
- How do you feel about epidurals or any pain medication?
- How long do you stay after the birth?
- Do you have experience with breastfeeding instruction?
- Do you offer any additional services, such as placenta encapsulation?
- Is it possible to read any reviews you might have?
- Do you also take pictures?

QUESTIONS TO ASK YOURSELF
(after the interviews)

- Did you feel as if she/he was really listening to you during the interview?
- Did you feel comfortable with her/him?
- Did she/he seem compassionate?
- Did she/he ask you any questions?
- Did you feel she/he was interested in you and what you want?
- Did she/he communicate well?
- Did she/he seem knowledgeable?
- Did her/his views on pregnancy, childbirth and care align with your own?
- Did she/he take the time to answer all of your questions or did you feel rushed?
- Was it easy to make the appointment with her/him?
- Did you click with her/him?
- Are they available around the time of your guess date?

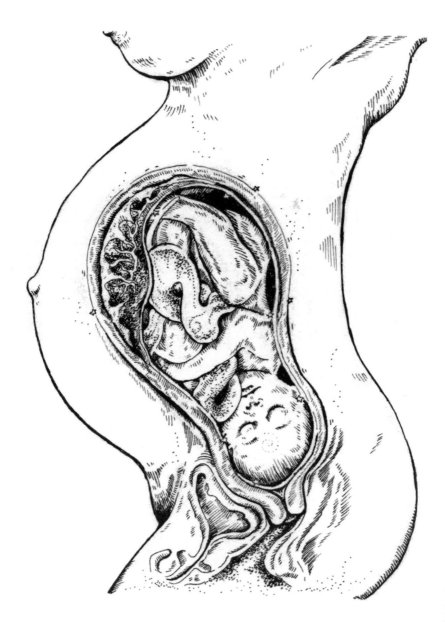

Nikki Scioscia

CHAPTER 6: ULTRASOUNDS

"Because ultrasound should only be used when medically indicated... For women with an uncomplicated pregnancy, an ultrasound is not a necessary part of prenatal care."
- AMERICAN PREGNANCY ASSOCIATION

"When enough women realize that birth is a time of great opportunity to get in touch with their true power, and when they are willing to assume responsibility for this, we will reclaim the power of birth and help move technology where it belongs— in the service of birthing women, not their master."
- CHRISTIANE NORTHRUP

"Many mothers have reported babies kicking intensively when receiving ultrasound. It is well known that animals such as whales and dolphins react negatively to the use of underwater Doppler and on scans babies are sometimes seen covering their ears."
- JOHN WILKS
Choices in Pregnancy & Childbirth

ULTRASOUNDS HAVE A PLACE in pregnancy. But the frequency, both in terms of how often as well as the sound, has become another part of routine care that is expensive, excessive, and as you will read, possibly detrimental. It is time for all of us to stop blindly accepting and instead ignite our inquisition and our will. I write this chapter intending to share information that mothers should know, so they can make educated decisions and requests, and question the routine and normalized practices that may not be rooted in necessity. Parents deserve to know potential adverse effects. For instance, if a doctor orders an ultrasound just to check the position of the baby, the mother can decline and ask that the position be felt with their hands instead. If a doctor orders an ultrasound just to see the growth of the baby, the mother can request that she/he measure her belly instead.

In 2001, 67% of pregnant women had at least one ultrasound.
In 2009, 99.8% of pregnant women had an average of three ultrasounds.
In 2019, pregnant women have an average of 5 ultrasounds.

Ultrasounds became a standard protocol for pregnant mothers about 40 years ago. Fetuses today are exposed to an unprecedented amount of scans, not just in frequency, but length and intensity. According to the American Congress of Obstetricians and Gynecologists (ACOG), a woman "should have at least one standard exam, usually performed at 18–22 weeks of pregnancy." They recommend 1–2 scans for a low-risk pregnancy, and it is estimated that 75 percent of all pregnancies are considered low-risk.

It is not uncommon for some mothers to get up to 12 ultrasounds in one pregnancy. Doctors might even order one per week from 34 weeks on, simply to determine the position of the baby; the skill of using their hands and/or a fetoscope is waning as technology takes over. Ultrasounds are performed earlier and later in pregnancy, more often, with higher intensity or acoustic output and longer duration, by technicians who may or may not be adequately trained or have any medical background.

There is a lot of money being made on women having more and more ultrasounds. Some doctors have an ultrasound machine in their office and use it whenever they want, without even filing an insurance claim. Scans are not always covered by insurance; they may only cover them if it is medically necessary, or partially cover them, or there may be a limit. Even if the insurance company covers the procedure, the mother may be responsible for a co-pay of up to $50 or more. For patients not covered by health insurance, one abdominal ultrasound typically costs $200–$650 or more, depending on the provider and geographic region, with a national average of $390, according to NewChoiceHealth.com. Ultrasounds and their price range listed below:

Fetal Biophysical Profile Cost Average	$350–$4200
Pregnant Ultrasound Cost Average	$270–$2400
Ultrasound of Fetus Cost Average	$290–$4000
Ultrasound of the Uterus Cost Average	$220–$4100

WHAT IS AN ULTRASOUND?

An ultrasound is a procedure that uses high-frequency sound waves to scan a woman's abdomen and pelvic cavity, creating a picture (sonogram) of the baby and placenta. Although the terms ultrasound and sonogram are technically different, they are used interchangeably and refer to the same exam.

HOW IS AN ULTRASOUND PERFORMED?

The traditional procedure involves slathering gel on the abdomen to work as a conductor for sound waves. The technician uses a transducer to produce sound waves into the uterus, which then bounce off bones and tissue, and return to the transducer to create a black and white image of the fetus.

SEVEN DIFFERENT TYPES:
(from AmericanPregnancy.org)

Transvaginal Scans: Specially designed probe transducers used inside the vagina to generate sonogram images. Most often used during the early stages of pregnancy.

Standard Ultrasound: A traditional ultrasound exam that uses a transducer over the abdomen to generate 2-Dimensional images of the developing fetus.

Advanced Ultrasound: This exam is similar to the standard ultrasound, but targets a suspected problem and uses more sophisticated equipment.

Doppler Ultrasound: This imaging procedure measures slight changes in the frequency of the ultrasound waves as they bounce off moving objects, such as blood cells.

3-D Ultrasound: Uses specially designed probes and software to generate 3-Dimensional images of the developing fetus.

4-D or Dynamic 3-D Ultrasound: Uses specially designed scanners to look at the face and movements of the baby prior to delivery.

Fetal Echocardiography: Uses ultrasound waves to assess the baby's heart anatomy and function. This is used to help assess suspected congenital heart defects.

WHY IS IT DONE?

FIRST TRIMESTER: (weeks 1–12)
- Evaluate the presence, size, number, and location of the pregnancy
- Confirm heartbeat
- Estimate the gestational age/ Assess abnormal gestation
- Confirm molar or ectopic pregnancies

SECOND TRIMESTER: (weeks 13–26)
- Structural abnormalities
- Confirm multiples pregnancy
- Verify growth, confirm intrauterine death,
- Identify excessive or reduced levels of amniotic fluid
- Evaluation of fetal well-being,
- Diagnose fetal malformation
  » Weeks 13–14 for characteristics of potential Down syndrome
  » Weeks 18–20 for congenital malformations

THIRD TRIMESTER: (weeks 27–end of pregnancy)
- Identify placental location
- Confirm intrauterine death
- Assess fetal presentation, observe fetal movements
- Identify uterine and pelvic abnormalities of the mother

ALTERNATIVE METHODS:
- Confirm pregnancy: pregnancy test (98% accurate), blood test
- Confirm heartbeat: use a fetoscope (usually audible by about 20 weeks)
- Estimate gestational age: date of conception, hormone levels in the mother's blood, date of the last menstrual period

- Verify growth: mother lies down and care provider measures from the top of the pubic bone to the top of the uterus with a tape measure (fundal height)
- Evaluation of fetal well being: ask mother if she feels movement
- Assess fetal presentation: feel the mother's belly to see where the buttocks, head, and or feet are; also find heartbeat location with a fetoscope

VALID MEDICAL REASONS

Fetal ultrasound is not recommended for finding out a baby's gender, or for entertainment. There are places today that offer packages to "bond with the baby" via HD Live, 3d or 4d viewing, including a room to invite family and friends. In a Consumer Update, revised in December 2014, the U.S. Food and Drug Administration said it "strongly discourages" the use of fetal ultrasound imaging and Doppler fetal ultrasound heartbeat monitors for non-medical reasons, like creating "keepsake images and videos." The FDA has been weighing in on the trend since 2008, and the update is meant to promote "the safe and prudent use of ultrasound" by trained and skilled operators.

The World Health Organization, the FDA, the American Pregnancy Association, the American College of Obstetrics and Gynecology all use similar language that states scans be done when "medically necessary" or "medically indicated" or "for medical reasons." Some of the reasons additional ultrasounds may be necessary:

- There are signs that the fetus is not growing well
- Mother has not felt the baby move recently
- Mother has had spotting during pregnancy
- "Due" date has passed and doctors want to check to see if the baby is okay
- There are known or suspected fetal anatomic abnormalities
- Mother is obese, which increases the risk of stillbirth and preeclampsia
- Mother has high blood pressure, chronic hypertension, diabetes, or is HIV positive

WHEN DID ULTRASOUNDS BECOME ROUTINE?

Ultrasound was first used for clinical purposes in 1956 in Glasgow, Scotland. Obstetrician Ian Donald and engineer Tom Brown developed the prototype systems based on an instrument used to detect industrial flaws in ships. They perfected its clinical use and by the late 1950s, ultrasounds were routinely used in Glasgow hospitals. It became popular in British hospitals in 1970, and it was the late 1970s before it became widely used in American hospitals." (source: "Imaging and Imagining the Fetus: The Development of Obstetric Ultrasound" (The Johns Hopkins University Press, 2013), Malcolm Nicolson and John Fleming) My mother birthed me in 1978, my brother in 1975, sister in 1974, and she did not have one ultrasound with any of us.

WHY THE INCREASE IN ULTRASOUND EXPOSURE?

It is a routine practice, therefore mothers consider it part of the experience of pregnancy, and likely don't know much about them, other than having seen the classic black and white image from their friends, sisters, etc. It is the "seeing is believing" mentality. The feeling of the baby goes from subtle to gross, and we are accustomed to seeing the gross before the subtle.

We human beings have a difficult time with mystery. Yes, the ability to see inside the uterus can have benefit, but it has become another way to play on the fears of the parents. If you don't look, you won't know. Sometimes it can seem there is a search for problems: the baby is measuring too big or too small, there is too much fluid, too little fluid, not enough growth, advanced maternal age, etc. I have heard from mothers that were told there is a risk for something, but "nothing to worry about." Easier said than done. From then on, the mother was much more reluctant to decline any of the doctors orders. It is very common for mothers to be told things like, "I want you to be delivered by 39 weeks," or "We will want to induce you at 40 weeks," or "You will have to have a C-section," because of an ultrasound.

DO MORE SCANS IMPROVE OUTCOME?

The frequency of ultrasounds has drastically increased without evidence to support why. There have been studies over the years to debunk the persuading promise that having more ultrasounds will improve the health of the baby or fetal outcomes. One study of 15,151 pregnant women, by the RADIUS

Study Group, published in the *New England Journal of Medicine*, was conducted by a team of six researchers over four years and compared pregnant women who received two scans to pregnant women who received scans only when some other medical indication suggested an ultrasound was necessary.

The results showed no difference in fetal outcomes. The authors concluded that among low-risk pregnant women ultrasound screening does not improve perinatal outcome. Even when the ultrasound uncovered abnormalities, the fetal survival rate was the same in both groups. What the authors found was that routine ultrasounds led to more expensive prenatal care, adding over $1 billion to the cost of caring for pregnant women in America each year.

Ultrasound can be used to diagnose potentially fatal or debilitating abnormalities in the fetus, playing a role in decisions to terminate or continue a pregnancy. For instance, in a midterm scan, parents may find out about untreatable issues such as heart and brain abnormalities, where the baby may or may not make it to term, or the mother is at high risk to carry the child. If abnormalities do appear in a scan, an MRI and/or an echocardiogram may be recommended to help doctors confirm and offer advice to parents. "Ultrasound may have a limited role in detection of a treatable indication, which Judy Cohain CNM stated, "only includes spina bifida—a birth defect where there is incomplete closing of the backbone and membranes around the spinal cord, diaphragmatic anomaly, twin-twin transfusion syndrome, bladder obstructions, and tumors that develop at the base of the coccyx."

Ultrasound can create a lot of stress and anxiety in the mother if, for instance, a shadow appears around the baby's heart, but then disappears in the subsequent scans. Many abnormalities found in the fetus can turn out to be an incorrect diagnosis. A UK survey showed that, for one in 200 babies aborted for major abnormalities, the diagnosis on post-mortem was less severe than predicted by ultrasound. Sometimes the ultrasound findings are not easily construed and the outcome for the baby is unknown. Dr. Sarah Buckley, author of a wonderful article titled "Ultrasounds Scans, Cause for Concern," chose not to receive them with her four children, and offers the following thoughts, "To my mind, ultrasound also represents yet another way in which the deep internal knowledge that a mother has of her body and her baby is made secondary to technological information that comes from an 'expert' using a machine. Thus the 'cult of the expert' is imprinted from the earliest weeks of life. Furthermore, by treating the baby as a separate being, ultrasound artificially splits mother from baby well before this is a physiological or psychic reality. This further emphasizes our cultures favoring of individualism over mutuality and sets the scene for possible- but to my mind artificial- conflicts of interest between mother and baby in pregnancy, birth and parenting."

In some East Asian countries, ultrasound is used to determine gender of the baby, and since a boy is often deemed more desirable, the girl might be aborted.

AT RISK PREGNANCIES

In higher-risk pregnancies (advanced maternal age, metabolic syndromes, complications), ultrasound is applied more frequently, thereby exposing the fetus (who may be more vulnerable) to the potential side effects more often.

> "Researchers in the Timing of Serial Ultrasound In At-Risk Pregnancies: A Randomized Controlled Trial (SUN Trial) conducted a randomized controlled study in which they enrolled approximately 200 women with conditions that can affect a baby's growth or the amount of amniotic fluid around it. The women were randomly divided into two groups: one received ultrasounds every four weeks while the other received them twice as often (every two weeks). The study then evaluated the differences in frequency of problems that were discovered, such as abnormal growth, low fluid levels, or other complications that might prompt early delivery. The result was a little surprising. In the end, researchers concluded that more frequent ultrasounds did not identify problems more frequently during the third trimester of complex pregnancies." – Robyn Horsager-Boehrer, M.D. Obstetrics & Gynecology, Are More Ultrasounds Better in Complicated Pregnancy?, May 8, 2018

WHO PROVIDES THE MACHINES?

Given the lack of evidence for ultrasonography's role in improving pregnancy and birth outcomes, one might ask why might The International Society of Ultrasound in Obstetrics and Gynecology (ISUOG) unilaterally recommends that all pregnant women have routine obstetric ultrasounds? One potential reason may be their partnership with the leading global obstetric technology companies, such as GE Healthcare, Phillips, Samsung Medison, Toshiba, and Siemens. So those who are recommending the ultrasounds profit with the companies providing the technology.

The use of Doppler ultrasound to monitor the baby's heartbeat has increased. According to the 2006 Cochrane Database of Systematic Reviews, "routine Doppler ultrasound in pregnancy does not have health benefits for women or babies and may do some harm."

HOW TO HEAR THE BABY'S HEARTBEAT & DETERMINE FETAL POSITIONING?

There is an instrument called a Pinard horn, invented by Dr. Adolphe Pinard, a French obstetrician, during the 19th century. Pinard was an early supporter of advancements in prenatal care, including closer fetal health monitoring. It is a type of stethoscope, sometimes called a "fetoscope." It functions similarly to an ear trumpet by amplifying sound. The wide end of the horn is held against the pregnant woman's belly, while the doctor, nurse, midwife or partner listens through the other end. A Pinard horn can also be used to determine the position of the fetus and is considered more precise than a Doppler device for this purpose. A Doppler device detects a heart tone farther away from the location of origin. A Pinard horn must be pressed to a location very close to the fetal heart in order to detect it, providing a more accurate indication of fetal position.

Midwives and others worldwide continue to use fetoscopes to listen to fetal heart tones. The United States is one of the few countries where the Doppler has replaced the fetoscope. Though there are many types of fetoscopes available, the most commonly used is the "Allen Type," where you place the ends in your ears, an oval piece on the forehead, and the circular piece on the mother's belly. Fetal heart tones can be detected as early as 18 weeks, but usually, a fetoscope is most effective after 22 weeks, which means the mother may have to wait a month longer to hear it, which in our culture may be challenging since we tend to want things as fast as we can get them! A heartbeat sound via a fetoscope is soft and far different than the amplified sound provided by a Doppler. When I had a required visit to an OBGYN, I requested she use a fetoscope instead of Doppler, to which she readily agreed; yet it took her a little while to go find it. When she returned, she laughed and said she had to pull it out of storage and dust it off, and commented that my midwife was probably much better at finding the heartbeat with it.

A doctor, nurse, or midwife can also use palpation to determine fetal position. A woman's intuition and consciousness of her body can often be enough to know the position of the baby, especially towards the final month. Movement of limbs is a good indication as to where they are. Belly Mapping is a three-step process for identifying a baby's position in the final months of pregnancy (Spinningbabies.com has info about this).

Only 5–7% of babies emerge directly in OP position (occiput posterior fetal position), which is when the back of baby's head is against the mother's back (i.e. face upwards). The rest rotate in labor. Childbirth texts estimate 15–30% of babies are in OP position in labor. Midwife Jean Sutton in Optimal Fetal Positioning describes that 50% of babies tend toward a posterior presentation, which aims the top of the head into the pelvis in early labor.

ARE ULTRASOUNDS SAFE?

Ultrasound technology was grandfathered into FDA clearance in 1976, assuming that it was safe, and several years later, studies on the technology ceased. Epidemiologic studies (who, when, where, patterns and determinants of health and disease) of ultrasound safety were conducted before 1992 and would have been representative of significantly less cumulative epigenetic burden to the fetus (relating to or arising from nongenetic influences on gene expression) as they predated changes to the childhood vaccination program and the flooding of diets with genetically modified foods—all of which may synergize in a vulnerable child to contribute to chronic neurodevelopmental problems.

In 1992 the FDA approved an eight-fold increase in the potential acoustical output of ultrasound equipment. In several decades, ultrasound technology has increased in peak exposure and intensity; the total radiant power of all wavelengths passing from all incident directions onto an infinitesimally small area has gone from a maximum of 46 mW/cm2 to 720 mW/cm2 (milliwatts per square centimeter). I repeat—46 to 720.

Newer machines employ significantly stronger signals, are not standardized by any regulations, are frequently defective, are largely unstudied, and are without federal requirements for operator training. The operators may have no medical background of adequate training.

ELEVATED SOUND & TEMPERATURE

The following information appeared in a 2006 article titled "Questions about Prenatal Ultrasound and the Alarming Increase in Autism" by Caroline Rodgers, in *Midwifery Today* magazine. The full article can be read at MidwiferyToday.com.

"One challenge that ultrasound operators face is keeping the transducer positioned over the part of the fetus the operator is trying to visualize. When fetuses move away from the stream of high-frequency sound waves, they may be feeling vibrations, heat or both. As the FDA warned in 2004, "ultrasound is a form of energy, and even at low levels, laboratory studies have shown it can produce physical effect in tissue, such as jarring vibrations and a rise in temperature." This is consistent with research conducted in 2001 in which an ultrasound transducer aimed directly at a miniature hydrophone placed in a woman's uterus recorded sound "as loud as a subway train coming into the station."

Across mammalian species, elevated maternal or fetal body temperatures have been shown to result in birth defects in offspring. An extensive review of literature on maternal hyperthermia in a range of mammals found that "central nervous system (CNS) defects appear to be the most common consequence of hyperthermia in all species, and cell death or delay in proliferation of neuroblasts [embryonic cells that develop into nerve cells] is believed to be one major explanation for these effects."

A study reported in the *Journal of the American Medical Association (JAMA)* found that "women who used hot tubs or saunas during early pregnancy face up to triple the risk of bearing babies with spina bifida or brain defects." Hot tubs and baths present greater dangers than other heat therapies such as saunas and steam rooms because the immersion in water foils the body's attempt to cool off via perspiration, in much the same way fetuses cannot escape elevated temperatures in the womb.

An individual's body temperature varies throughout the day due to various factors such as circadian rhythms, hormone fluctuations and physical exertion. While people may have up to 1.5° F in each direction of what is considered a "normal" core temperature, the overall average among people is 98.6° F. An increase of only 1.4° F to 100° F can cause headaches, body aches and fatigue, enough to get the individual excused from work. A temperature of 107° F can cause brain damage or death.

A core temperature of about 98.6° F is important because that is the point at which many important enzyme reactions occur. Temperature affects the actual shape of the proteins that create enzymes, and improperly shaped proteins are unable to do their jobs correctly. As factors such as the amount of heat or duration of exposure increase, enzyme reactions become less efficient until they are permanently inactivated, unable to function correctly even if the temperature returns to normal.

Because temperature is critical to proper enzyme reactions, the body has built-in methods to regulate its core temperature. For instance, when it is too low, shivering warms it up; when it is too high, sweating wicks off the heat. For obvious reasons, fetuses cannot cool off by sweating. However, they have another defense against temperature increases: Each cell contains something called heat shock (HS) proteins that temporarily stop the formation of enzymes when temperatures reach dangerously high levels.

Complicating the issue is the fact that ultrasound heats bone at a different rate than muscle, soft tissue or amniotic fluid. Further, as bones calcify, they absorb and retain more heat. During the third trimester, the baby's skull can heat up 50 times faster than its surrounding tissue, subjecting parts of the brain that are close to the skull to secondary heat that can continue after the ultrasound exam has concluded.

Elevated temperatures that might only temporarily affect the mother can have devastating effects on a developing embryo. A 1998 article in the medical journal *Cell Stress & Chaperones* (an integrative journal of stress biology and medicine) reported that, "the HS response is inducible in early embryonic life but it fails to protect embryos against damage at certain stages of development." The authors noted, "With activation of the HS response, normal protein synthesis is suspended…but survival is achieved at the expense of normal development."(22)

〰

In 1984, when the National Institutes of Health held a conference assessing ultrasound risks, it reported that when birth defects occurred, the acoustic output was usually high enough to cause considerable heat. Although the NIH has since stated that the report "is no longer viewed…as guidance for current medical practice," the facts remain unchanged.

NEURODEVELOPMENT

A Cornell University team of researchers proved in 2001 that brain development proceeds in the same manner "across many mammalian species, including human infants," and found "95 neural developmental milestones" that helped identify the sequence of brain growth in different species. If experiments show that elevated heat caused by ultrasound damages fetal brains in rats and other mammals, it seems logical that it could harm human brains too.

Jim West, who has compiled the largest human ultrasound studies, notated in *50 Human Studies, in Utero, Conducted in Modern China, Indicate Extreme Risk for Prenatal Ultrasound: A New Bibliography*, says, "Unknown to Western scientists, the hazards of ultrasound have been confirmed in China since the late 1980s, where thousands of women, volunteering for abortion, thousands of maternal-fetal pairs, were exposed to carefully controlled diagnostic ultrasound and the abortive matter then analyzed via laboratory techniques. The data from about 65 studies involving 100 scientists and 2,700 mother-fetal pairs, employed electron microscopy, flow cytometry, and various biochemical analysis (immuno- and histo-) with results compared against those of sham-exposed pregnant women (exposed at zero intensity). Assessing brain, kidney, cornea, chorionic villi and the immune system, researchers determined the amount of ultrasound exposure required to produce damage to the human fetus to be very low."

West cites Professor Ruo Feng, who reviewed many of the studies, and stipulated, "Routine ultrasound be avoided. Only if there were exceptional medical indications should ultrasound be allowed, and at minimum intensity. Sessions should be very brief, no more than 3 minutes, 5 minutes at most. Multiple sessions should be avoided because hazards are cumulative. Human studies had found sensitive organs damaged at 1-minute exposure." Ruo Feng is the editor of The Chinese Journal of Ultrasound in Medicine and Biology, member of the World Federation of Ultrasound in Medicine and Biology, and Professor at The Institute of Acoustics at Nanjing University.

The risks to the baby are potentially higher due to the higher acoustic output required for high-definition images, a potentially long session—as technicians hunt for suitable images—along with factors such as cavitation (a bubbling effect caused by ultrasound that can damage cells) make the impact of ultrasound uncertain even in expert hands.

According to the peer-reviewed medical resource, UpToDate: "Spectral Doppler ultrasound uses higher energy and focuses the acoustic energy that is created on a much smaller volume of tissue than typical 2D imaging does, and can result in changes in tissue temperature, especially at bone-tissue interfaces. For this reason, Doppler ultrasound should be used with great care, especially early in pregnancy."

AUTISM

Autism Spectrum Disorder (ASD) is on the rise worldwide, not just the United States. In the UK, teachers report that 1 in 86 primary school children have special needs related to ASD. The causes of autism have been linked to vaccines, genetics, immunological disorders, environmental toxins, and maternal infections. "Although proponents point out that ultrasound has been used in obstetrics for 50 years and early studies indicated it was safe for both mother and child, enough research has implicated it in neurodevelopmental disorders to warrant serious attention." (Rodgers) There are many studies, too many to discuss here. If you care to explore this subject further, please do so.

In May 2006, figures from the Centers for Disease Control (CDC) spawned a greater awareness of ASD, deeming it an "urgent public health issue." Only 12 years prior, autism (characterized by a range of learning and social impairments) was so rare that it occurred in just one in 10,000 births. In 2006, it was reported to occur in one in 166 children. It has continued rising and the CDC's latest statistics show that in 2014, in America, 1 in 59 children had a diagnosis by age 8.

That bears repeating.

In 1994, 1 in 10,000 children.

In 2006, 1 in 166 children.

In 2014, 1 in 59 children.

In August 2006, the chair of Yale's School of Medicine Department of Neurobiology announced the results of a study in which pregnant mice underwent various durations of ultrasound. The brains of the offspring showed damage consistent with that found in the brains of people with autism. The research, funded by the National Institute of Neurological Disorders and Stroke, also implicated ultrasound in neurodevelopmental problems in children, such as dyslexia, epilepsy, mental retardation, and schizophrenia, and showed that damage to brain cells increased with longer exposures.

"Geneticists are trying to crack the DNA mysteries behind autism. Recently researchers linked two mutations of the same X chromosome gene to autism in two unrelated families, although they do not yet know at what stage these genes were damaged. Because sibling and twin studies show a higher prevalence of autism among children in families with one autistic child, geneticists expected to find inherited factors, but despite millions of dollars invested in the search, no clear explanation indicates that ASD is inherited. Since both twins are exposed to ultrasound at the same time, it stands to reason that if one twin were autistic, the other would have a high probability of being affected. But in both identical and fraternal twins, one twin could be more severely affected than the other if she or he were receiving more of the heat or sound waves. A 2002 study showed that simply being a twin substantially increased the likelihood of autism, making twinning a risk factor. Could this have to do with the practice of giving mothers with multiple gestations more ultrasounds than those expecting single births?" (Rodgers)

INCREASINGLY COMMON BIRTH DEFECTS

One of the most popular non-medical uses of ultrasound is to determine the baby's gender, increasing the energy directed at the sexual organs. There has been an increase in birth defects involving the genitals and urinary tract, which affects "as many as 1 in 10 babies," according to the March of Dimes, adding that "specific causes of most of these conditions is unknown." Another part of the body scrutinized by ultrasound technicians is the heart, where serious defects soared nearly 250 percent between 1989 and 1996. "The list of unexplained birth defects is not a short one, and in light of what is emerging about prenatal ultrasound, scientists should take another look at all recent trends, as well as the baffling 30% increase in premature births since 1981, now affecting one in every eight children, with many showing subsequent neurological damage." (Rodgers)

Just because a lifestyle and approach to health has become normalized does not make them best for our evolution. Antibiotics, processed foods, pesticides, industrial chemicals, vaccines, ultrasound, increased amounts of surgical births, formula feeding, don't necessarily contribute to a healthy child. Care providers, pediatricians, government, technology companies, play a huge role in influencing the health of the children, and parents' decisions. Our children deserve better. Pregnant mothers and their partners deserve honest and quality care and more transparency. If you choose to have a scan, have it done by a skillful and experienced operator. Tell them to make it as brief as possible. Request the least amount of intensity.

West and Feng quotes are from "The Risk of Exposure to Diagnostic Ultrasound in Postnatal Subjects Thermal Effects" by William D. O'Brien, Jr, PhD, Cheri X. Deng, PhD, et.al, J Ultrasound Med. 2008 Apr; 27(4): 517–540.

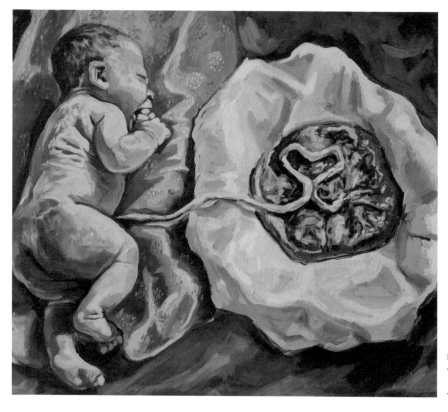

CHAPTER 7:
UMBILICAL CORD

"Another thing very injurious to the child, is the tying and cutting of the navel string too soon; which should always be left till the child has not only repeatedly breathed but till all pulsation in the cord ceases. As otherwise the child is much weaker than it ought to be, a portion of the blood being left in the placenta, which ought to have been in the child."
— ERASMUS DARWIN,
(Charles Darwin's grandfather) 1801

"It is common practice nowadays for the cord to be doubly clamped while the child is on the mother's abdomen and the scissors are handed to the parents to complete the job. Most mothers refuse, leaving it to the husband; some mothers recoil in horror, and if the cord is left intact, most mothers will not touch it. If they do, and especially if it is pulsating, the cord is treated as gently and tenderly as is a tiny finger or an ear of the child. New mothers are strongly inhibited from damaging the cord."
— DR. G. M. MORLEY

I HAVE HAD A belly button my entire life but haven't always known it as a mark of my umbilical cord. The cord was our lifeline. My son's is dried out, in the shape of a heart, in a plastic baggie in his baby book. I may eventually frame it. I think the cord is fascinating. Take a look at your belly button and see where yours once was. It is either cavernous or poking outward, and in some cases, there is no scar at all.

The umbilical cord is also called the navel string, birth cord, or funiculus umbilicus. In placental mammals, it is the conduit between the developing embryo and placenta. During prenatal development, the umbilical cord is physiologically and genetically part of the fetus. The umbilical cord develops from and contains remnants of the yolk sac and allantois. It forms by the 5th week of fetal development, replacing the yolk sac as the source of nutrients for the fetus. The cord is not directly connected to the mother's circulatory system, but instead joins the placenta, which transfers materials to and from the mother's blood without allowing direct mixing.

The umbilical cord in a full term baby is usually around 55 centimeters long and 2 centimeters in diameter. The diameter decreases rapidly within the placenta. An umbilical cord is considered short if it measures fewer than 35 centimeters in length.

In humans, the cord normally contains two arteries and one vein that are buried within a gelatinous substance called Wharton's jelly, which is mostly made of mucopolysaccharides. This jelly helps keep the cord free from knots and protected from blood vessel compression. The vein passively supplies the fetus with oxygenated, nutrient-rich blood from the placenta. The two arteries carry deoxygenated, nutrient-depleted blood from the fetus back to the placenta. Occasionally, one vein and only one artery is present in the umbilical cord, and is sometimes related to fetal abnormalities, but may also occur without accompanying problems. The blood flow through the umbilical cord is approximately 35 ml, about six teaspoons, at 20 weeks, and 240 ml, about 1 cup, at 40 weeks of gestation.

The umbilical cord enters the fetus via the abdomen, at the point which (after separation) will become the umbilicus (or navel). Within the fetus, the umbilical vein continues towards the liver, where it splits into two branches: one branch joins with the hepatic portal vein, which carries blood into the liver. The other branch bypasses the liver and flows into the inferior vena cava, which carries blood towards the heart. The two umbilical arteries branch from the internal iliac arteries, and pass on either side of the urinary bladder into the umbilical cord, completing the circuit back to the placenta.

The first few minutes of life are pretty important! All mammals switch from placental to lung breathing at birth by themselves and have done so for millions of years. Before birth, a large part of the fetal blood volume is circulating in the placenta, where it picks up its supply of oxygen and nutrients. Kind of like scuba gear, until the fetus becomes a neonate and takes its first deep breath. That moment sets in motion the massive transition from sending blood to the placenta for essentials to sending blood to the lungs.

The umbilical cord continues to carry the babies' blood back and forth from the placenta until nature sends signals that:

1. The lungs are working fine (high oxygen saturation)
2. Vital organs have enough blood flow (central venous pressure rises to that of healthy neonate)

After these signals are received, the fetal blood that is left in the placenta—about 40% of the newborn's total blood volume—is squeezed back to the fetus to fill the lungs (placental transfusion). The arteries and vein in the cord constrict, and their walls get swollen, thereby cutting off all blood flow. In humans, without drugs interfering, this "natural clamp" (loss of umbilical cord pulsations and no blood flowing through) occurs 1 to 6 minutes after birth; with drugs, the range is 1–20 minutes. Therefore, one minute, which is considered in most hospitals to be "delayed cord-cutting," is not enough.

Also know, that even though they may wait to cut the cord, they will likely still clamp it right away. I once watched a doctor, who promised delayed cord-cutting to the mother, clamp it immediately, cut it 45 seconds later, and then tug on it to try and pull the placenta out of the mother (to hurry up the process.) It was one of the first few births I attended as a doula. I learned that even if parents share their wishes with the caregiver beforehand, they must be reaffirmed, repeatedly, if necessary, during the process, in order to ensure they are adhered to.

> "...Immediate cord clamping is clearly identified as a cause of newborn neurological (brain) injury ranging from neonatal death through cerebral palsy to mental retardation and behavioral disorders. Immediate cord clamping has become increasingly common in obstetrical practice over the past 20 years; today, rates of behavioral disorders (*e.g.*, ADD/ADHD) and developmental disorders (*e.g.*, autism, Asperger's, etc) continue to climb and are not uncommon in grade school." – Dr. George M. Morley

> "Delaying clamping the umbilical cord for a slightly longer period of time allows more umbilical cord blood volume to

transfer to the infant and, with that critical period extended, many good physiological "gifts" are transferred through 'nature's first stem cell transplant' occurring at birth." (Tolosa and Park, et. al, *Journal of Cellular and Molecular Medicine*, 2010)

Watch Penny Simkin's "Delayed Cord Clamping" video on youtube.

WHY IS IT A STANDARD PRACTICE TO CUT THE UMBILICAL CORD IMMEDIATELY AFTER A BABY IS BORN? WHY IS IT CUT AT ALL? WHEN DID THIS BEGIN?

Until the 1960s, doctors generally waited until the umbilical cord pulsations stopped before clamping and cutting the cord (several minutes). But then things changed, and they started clamping the cord "immediately," which means 10–30 seconds after birth —no placental transfusion and no waiting for blood to return to the baby before clamping.

The Royal College of Obstetricians and Gynecologists states, "Active management of the third stage of labor [of which early clamping is a pillar] became part of clinical practice in the 1960s, accompanying the widespread introduction of oxytocin." In other words, the practice of cutting the umbilical cord began when doctors took up the habit of inducing labor with an artificial oxytocin drug. Because drugs and epidurals cross the placenta and adversely affect the infant, early clamping of the cord would be done, cutting off crucial oxygen to the baby. Therefore, they had to be quick in moving the infant (usually for resuscitation, go figure) to a warm environment, ready to intervene in the event of crises for transfer to the Neonatal ICU. They couldn't take the baby away while waiting for the placental/cord unit to stop delivering blood. I have wondered, when the mother is in the hospital setting, "Why not place/move the resuscitation table right next to the mother, so the cord doesn't have to get cut?" Or why not bring the tools to the baby on the mother's chest (oxygen, suction tools, etc.)?

A private market has developed for umbilical cord blood (available only if the cord is clamped early), which is an extremely rich source of stem cells. Also, cosmetic companies are keen to obtain human cord and placental tissue for use in their products.

WHY IS IT CUT AT ALL?

"When I am asked, "Why don't you cut babies' umbilical cords?" I say, "Isn't the real question: Why do you cut?" It's interesting that those of us on the path of nonviolence are being asked to justify our peaceful non-intervention, by the perpetrators of intemperate protocols." – Ibu Robin Lim, CPM

Cutting the cord is literally an amputation. Many who have cut the cord report it to be somewhat tough, like a finger or a toe.

RISKS OF EARLY CUTTING/CLAMPING:

- Hypovolemia, hypotension and shock (after all, the cord blood represents as much as 40% of infant's blood volume!)
- Hypoxia, especially if the neonate doesn't breathe well right away. Clamping the cord too early is like closing up the hose to your scuba tank before you reach the surface to breathe.
- Anemia is a condition that develops when your blood lacks enough healthy red blood cells or hemoglobin. It is the most common blood condition in the U.S.
- A combination of the above factors raises concern about brain damage.
- The premature loss of the richest source of stem cells (and of essential hormones and factors) in the neonate's body.

EXCERPT FROM ROBIN LIM, CPM:

"We need to not only protect the mother and the baby at birth, we need to protect the placenta, and we need to do that by not immediately clamping and cutting the umbilical cord. Because when you do that, you immediately deny the baby of 40–60% of his or her blood supply, which is still in the placenta with stem cells that are made in the placenta and move into the baby last. Without that full blood supply, your brain and all your organs are never fully innervated, so there is research showing that the leading cause for marginal retardation in the world today, which means people that are functioning normally but they are not functioning at full capacity. The leading cause of that is newborn anemia, which is caused by the immediate cutting and clamping of the umbilical cord. Remember, the clamping and cutting of the umbilical cord is a sterile procedure because it's inherently dangerous.

What happens the minute they clamp and cut that umbilical cord is they take that baby away from that mother, and that is the time of most profound learning. In that time when bonding is most important, that baby is learning separation, anxiety, fear, abandonment. And what does that come down to? "I'm going to die. The blood that was coming from my placenta that was oxygenating my body and my brain, that was making it so that I could actually breathe without my lungs which aren't activated yet." The heart is changing in those first moments of life. The way we absorbed oxygen into the bloodstream was dependent on the placenta. Now that the placenta has been clamped, we don't get that oxygenated blood anymore before our heart has made the exchange and our lungs are able to fill with air. That first breath, you have this incredible trauma, and without words you know that you are going to die. There is actually no reason to cut the cord and every reason not to. The World Health Organization has said that the immediate clamping and cutting of the umbilical cord is a protocol that needs to be justified. I don't see any justification. When the baby is premature, that is the one time that pediatricians wait, and even milk the cord toward the baby before the cutting to make sure to push the blood and the stem cells towards the baby."

BENEFITS OF DELAYED CORD CUTTING
- Higher birth weight, increased oxygen levels and nutrients
- Increased blood volume (32%)
- Increased red blood cells, stem cells and immune cells
- Increased iron stores, decreased risk for anemia (50%)

THE TREND OF BANKING CORD BLOOD
In the past couple of decades, it has become popular to bank the remaining blood left in the cord after it's cut (when not allowed time to transfer to the

baby). It is now a multi billion-dollar industry. There are 3 types of banks: private, public, and direct donation. The typical volume of cord blood collected is about 1.5–3 ounces.

Because the blood has stem cells, it is considered a precious resource. The American Medical Association recommends against storing cord blood, because the benefits are too remote to justify the costs. ALSO, IF IT IS A PRECIOUS RESOURCE, THEN WHY NOT GIVE IT TO THE BABY WHO'S IT IS?

> "We must be very clear. This blood is not "cord" blood, it is baby's blood! When we ask mothers to give away cord blood, they are under an illusion. This blood belongs to the baby, not the umbilical cord." – Robin Lim, CPM

CONS OF BANKING BLOOD

- The baby does not receive the blood they are entitled to and need!
- Collecting an insufficient volume of cord blood occurs in about half or more cases of cord blood collection.
- Cord blood collection includes limited cell doses (due to the small amount of cord blood) and quality control (issues due to the required storage).
- The chance of privately banked cord blood ever being used by your child is meager, currently less than 0.04%, according to the American Society for Blood and Marrow Transplantation.
- Contamination of the stem blood cells is possible.
- Collection and storage costs at private cord blood banks are high. The cost to bank blood ranges from $200–$10,000, with a $150–$300 annual fee. Some facilities have been shut down due to unsanitary conditions, dirty storage, leaky blood samples, etc. Stem cell transplant using an individual's own cord blood cannot be used for genetic disorders such as sickle cell disease, childhood cancer, or leukemia, because the genetic mutations that cause the disorders are present in their cord blood.

CORD BURNING INSTEAD OF CUTTING

The umbilicus is the entryway to all abdominal organs. It is the core. In traditional Chinese medicine, it is believed that the placenta holds the Ch'i (life force) of the baby. By heating the umbilical cord, the Ch'i goes to the baby, who is, therefore, "warmed" by this energy. Cord burning not only provides this warm energy, but it will reduce the risk of bleeding and chance of infection. You are warming the baby's digestion process, which will reduce the tendency for jaundice, as well as increasing the baby's nursing success.

A CORD BURNING TECHNIQUE:

Mother can be holding the baby. Cover a piece of cardboard with tinfoil. Make a slit/notch for the cord to slide into, creating a barrier between flames and baby. Hold two lit candles on either side of the cord and hold a bowl or wooden box underneath to catch the wax. Gradually, as the cord becomes thinner with burning, twist it gently with loving hands until it burns through completely. Within about 10 minutes, the entire process is complete, and the cord detaches.

WHAT IS A LOTUS BIRTH?

Jane Goodall reported in her book, In the Shadow of Man, that in her long observation of chimpanzees in the wild, they did not sever the umbilical cords of their babies. They participate in what is called "Lotus Birth," which entails leaving the umbilical cord intact until it naturally falls off of the baby's naval. Traditionally, among the Hopis, it is believed that the first humans were born from the womb of the Earth Mother, attached to her placenta by the umbilical cord. The Earth Mother's placenta was said to be like a tribe or community that nourishes its children. Even the early pioneers of America were said to have practiced umbilical non-severance to prevent infection from the open wound of a cut cord.

The lotus flower represents beauty, fertility, prosperity, spirituality, and eternity. In Buddhism, the lotus is known to be associated with purity, spiritual awakening, and faithfulness. The flower is pure as it can emerge from murky waters in the morning and be perfectly clean. The lotus is a sign of rebirth.

"If we think of a human life as a lotus plant: the placenta is the root, the cord is the stem and the baby the flower/fruit, perhaps, by watering this root in our hearts, some sense can be made of our lives. By nurturing where we come from, we may find clues as to where we are going. On this ailing planet, in our troubled times, may we embrace our origins and nourish our potential, to light our way safely home." – Sunni Karll

Not only is the baby immediately separated from the placenta, in most American hospitals, it is standard procedure to separate the baby from the mother just minutes after birth. American babies routinely have their umbilical cords clamped seconds after birth, cut a minute or less later, are given antibiotic ointment for their eyes to protect against venereal disease, a vitamin K shot in their thigh to avoid blood clotting disorders, and a hepatitis B vaccine. Though the numbers are declining, the majority of American baby boys will also have their penis mutilated, aka circumcised, within a day of being born. So healthy newborns are taken from their mother, sometimes without any skin to skin contact. Poked, prodded, shot, cut, and often not brought back for many minutes, which to a baby (and the mother) is a long time. Does a healthy newborn baby need so much medical intervention in the first few hours of her life?

For more on Lotus Birth, read the book *Sacred Birthing, Birthing a New Humanity* by Sunni Karll. See Placenta Chapter for how to preserve placenta while waiting for the cord to fall off.

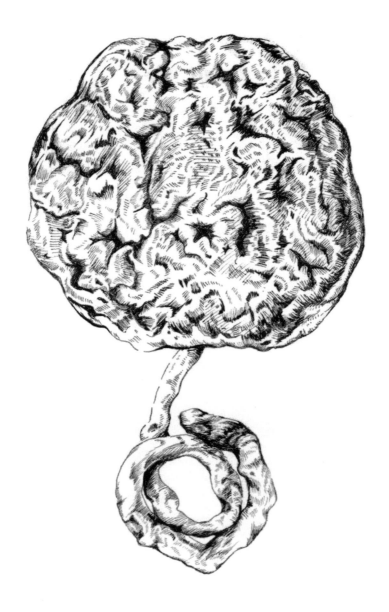

Nikki Scioscia

CHAPTER 8: PLACENTA

"The root of your origin, a miraculous organ that shares and protects your life. It is the conductor that unites you with your mother and serves as the control panel of the womb-ship that sustains you until you are born. It was conceived at the moment of your genesis. Your placenta is genetically identical to you. Though you share some of your parents' genetic identity, unless you have an identical twin, no one, except your placenta, has ever been so perfectly, exactly you."
- ROBIN LIM, Renowned Midwife, Author

"As mammals, we reproduce sexually, and sex is the reddest, hottest tile in the mosaic of our earthly lives. The placenta is at the epicenter of this miracle. Herstorically, our creation stories tell of the Earth Mother birthing the world: her amniotic fluid became the oceans, the placenta became the Tree of Life. This demonstrates how essential the placenta is to our survival and how embedded it is in our psyche."
- FROM *Placenta, The Forgotten Chakra*

BIRTHDAYS CONJURE UP THE image of a cake. Where did that start? Placenta is the circular shaped uterine "cake." The mother grows an entire organ that she will then birth after the baby. We would not exist without our placenta having been with us in the womb. If you research the origin of birthday cakes, you'll see a reference to Greece (plakuos=flat cake) and the German celebration Kinderfeste (the word for placenta is Mutterkuchen=mother cake). Ancient Greeks baked moon-shaped cakes to offer to the moon goddess Artemis, decorating them with lit candles to shine. A woman's moon cycle is how a baby manifests. So when we eat cake on our birthdays, it is a shout out to the moon, and to the very first "cake" in our life that fed us! If anyone has ever said to you, "You can't have your cake and eat it too," well, actually—you can. Read on.

New life only works because of the placenta. The placenta is crucial to the development of the embryo and fetus. In some traditions, the placenta is considered your angel, the spirit of it remaining with you from conception until the death of your body. Yet, in our modern culture, most of us know none to little about the placenta. I sure didn't before becoming pregnant. The National Institute of Child Health and Human Development calls the placenta, "the least understood human organ and arguably one of the more important, not only for the health of a woman and her fetus during pregnancy but also for the lifelong health of both."

Most hospitals in the west today dispose of the babies' placentas, tossing them out as mere medical waste.

The placenta is an organ that develops wherever the fertilized egg embeds in the uterus, after its journey along the fallopian tube. This organ provides oxygen and nutrients to the growing baby and removes waste products from the baby's blood. The placenta attaches to the wall of the uterus, and the baby's umbilical cord arises from it. The placenta can be situated anywhere on the surface of the uterus. An anterior placenta means the placenta positioning is on the front wall. But most of the time, a fertilized egg situates itself in the posterior wall of the uterus, the part closest to the spine, which is where the placenta eventually develops.

An Excerpt from *Placenta, The Forgotten Chakra* by Robin Lim

"Human beings are extremely dynamic systems, and our survival hinges on the strength of our individual immune systems. The placenta is the commander-in-chief of the baby's immune system during embryonic development. Thus, we must protect our offspring's placentas by being gentle during the transition of birth, to give our children the best possible start and protect the very foundation of their immune systems. What mother eats, drinks, feels, and experiences in her environment has an impact on the offspring's future health intelligence and entire genetic manifestation. All of this impacts the gestating child and will radiate out to her future generations. The conduit between mother's gestalt of experiences is the umbilical cord, and the placenta is the organ of synthesis."

TWO SIDES OF THE PLACENTA

MATERNAL SIDE

The maternal side has a spongy surface that looks like meat, attaches to the interior wall of the uterus, and gathers from the mother's blood stream precisely what the baby needs in the moment. The intelligence of the placenta sifts through all nutrients, choosing specific amounts of each vitamin or substance needed and draws it into the baby's bloodstream.

PLACENTA FUN FACTS
- Weighs 1 pound (or roughly 1/6 of the newborn's weight)
- Comes from the German meaning 'of mother's bread'

FETAL SIDE

The fetal side is smooth and glossy, and called the tree of life, with a beautiful silvery tree trunk of the umbilical cord and the branches or root system of veins and arteries. It is no surprise that our genealogy also uses this name. The placenta knows the family tree from the beginning of time and preserves the accumulation of cultural wisdom of each being within it. Our wisdom lies in our cells, bones, blood, body, and makes up generations to come.

From the beginning of the third month of pregnancy, the fetus and mother maintain completely separate blood systems, which is another miracle of the placenta—integrating mother and child while maintaining their integrity as individuals.

As the placenta develops and makes its rich cocktail of hormones, a normal, healthy pregnancy is typically maintained. The placenta secretes hormones that regulate uterine contractions, making the uterus a comfortable cocoon in which the baby can develop. These hormones also prepare the mother's body to lactate, which will be the baby's source of life postpartum. Thus, the placenta serves as a crucial life resource for the baby both within the womb and after birth.

BIRTHING THE PLACENTA

After the baby arrives, the placenta falls neatly away from the already shrinking uterine wall and birthed within 30 minutes after baby, although it may take up to 60 minutes. If after 60 minutes it has not yet come out, the care provider will assess the situation, and it may be necessary to manually extract it. If the extraction is not successful, and the entire organ or a portion of it remains inside (retained placenta), it can cause hemorrhage, and must be surgically removed. This is a very rare complication. Things to help the placenta's expulsion include: emptying the bladder, massaging the top of the uterus, moving to a seated, standing, or squatting position, and breastfeeding. Most traditional birth attendants know from experience that putting the baby skin to skin with the mother immediately after birth is the best way to stimulate the safe delivery of the placenta. Separation of mother and baby puts the mother at higher risk for postpartum hemorrhage. Dr. Sarah J Buckley states, "For the new mother, the third stage is a time of reaping the rewards of her labor. Mother Nature provides peak levels of oxytocin, the hormone of love, and endorphins, hormones of pleasure for both mother and baby. Skin-to-skin contact and the baby's first attempts to breastfeed further augment maternal oxytocin levels, strengthening the uterine contractions that will help the placenta to separate, and the uterus to contract down."

Many care providers are trained to catch the baby, give the mother a shot of Pitocin to help the uterus contract and prevent hemorrhage, clamp the cord, and steadily pull on it to get the placenta out swiftly. They will then massage the uterus to help it tighten and to cut off blood flow. Often this is done hastily to speed things along. Pulling on the umbilical cord, known as "controlled cord traction," carries a small risk of tearing the cord and of causing a rare but life-threatening condition called uterine inversion, in which the organ is pulled inside out or even out of the body.

DO MULTIPLES SHARE A PLACENTA?

A small number (1–2%) of identical twins share the same placenta and amniotic sac. Fraternal twins (from two separate fertilized eggs and sperms) each have their own placenta and their own amniotic sac. Fraternal triplets are three entirely separate and unique little pregnancies. Because of this, they will be enclosed in their own sacs and have their own placentas. Identical twins/triplets may or may not share the same amniotic sac, depending on how early the one fertilized egg divides into two.

IT'S YOUR ORGAN

You have grown this beautiful organ inside your body, which has fed your baby and is dense with nutrients. So how did the placenta, central to our survival and future well being, lose its significance and come to be considered garbage, medical waste, biohazard, tossed in the trash? Dr. Michel Odent, who specializes in Obstetrics, calls what has occurred in the 20th century "the industrialization of childbirth."

In 1994 it was discovered that approximately 360 tons of human placenta was being sold by hospitals annually to pharmaceutical companies for pharmaceuticals or use in the development of skin creams and hair products, under the guise of "research." That same year Britain banned the practice of collecting and marketing the placentas of unsuspecting citizens. A midwife friend of mine once worked at a hospital in the U.S. that sold placentas for $1 each to a shampoo company, but it stopped because of HIV.

In 2007, Poole Hospital, in the United Kingdom, sold the placentas of unwitting mothers to a biochemical company called Sigma-Aldrich, which then extracted the placentas' valuable proteins (like albumin) to sell to cosmetic scientists, some of whom were employed by the world's biggest cosmetic companies. The placenta is a rich raw material containing especially high levels of proteins and enzymes, like alkaline phosphatase and collagen, which are widely used in some cosmetics to stimulate skin growth, combat wrinkles, and strengthen hair. Poole Hospital insisted that the £5,000 it received for its placentas was a "donation" rather than a payment, and the money was used to buy medical equipment. Sigma-Aldrich advertises its human collagen at £1,215 for just half a gram and posts global pre-tax profits upwards of £195million.

Aside from the hospital's profiting, which was denounced by politicians and health policymakers alike, ethical concerns arose about how the obtainment of the mothers' consent. The mothers were asked to sign long-winded paperwork directly after giving birth that falsely stated the placenta would get used for medical research. One mother was outraged when she realized that the afterbirth of her daughter was given to a biochemical company, saying, "I was under the impression that my placenta would only be used for vital medical research—not that it may help make some skin cream or shampoo.

I feel violated. It feels like they stole it because it was all done on pretenses. It's from my body. I feel like they tricked it from me."

She was given a complex medical consent form to sign after giving birth. "They said my placenta would be used to help cure cancer research. They didn't mention anything else. I was elated having just given birth and just signed it." The consent form stated the placenta was for "research into... cancer, cystic fibrosis, Parkinson's disease and HIV/AIDS." Their potential use in cosmetic research is not mentioned, and mothers are not told that both the hospital and recipient of the placenta will profit from the trade. Sigma-Aldrich was asked to revise the information on the consent form and "be much more explicit about what the placentas are used for and mention the donation."

᠊᠊

Because in a hospital setting it is not normal protocol, if a mother wants to take the placenta home, she can tell the doctor during pregnancy, have it written in her chart, and let her partner/midwife/doula know so they can reinstate this wish come birthing time. She may be asked to sign a form called "Consent to Release Products of Childbirth." She can also request/provide a hospital release form to have on file/hand. After the placenta expulsion, remind them of this wish. The staff will put it in a plastic container with a label on it, and likely into a plastic bag. If taking the placenta home, it is wise to bring a small cooler bag along, to keep it cold (ask for ice from staff or doula will get for you). Some couples have smuggled it out in an ice bag, as there are certain cities and states where it is more challenging to procure your placenta. Some hospitals require a court order because it is considered transporting an organ. Some even require it be sent to a funeral home first!

A fairly publicized case that went to the courts was that of Anne Swanson, a new mother in Las Vegas, who, in 2007 after the birth of her daughter, requested to take her placenta home to be dried, ground into a powder and packed into capsules. The hospital refused to give it to her, and two weeks later, a county district court judge ordered the hospital to return it to Swanson. Remember, it is your babies' organ. You grew it, you own it, and it is not waste. It contains both their DNA and yours. You have a legal right to take it home.

For centuries, the practice of stimulating the placenta if a baby appears lifeless or does not breathe at birth has been practiced in India, Bangladesh and Burma. Warming the placenta (in a bowl of warm water) and/or massaging it will activate the prana (life force) of the child, which is stored in the placenta and passed gradually into the baby.

EATING THE PLACENTA

More than 4000 species of mammals consume their placenta. Humans are one of few mammals who do not eat their placenta. Except for camelids and marine mammals, all other mammals consume their afterbirth. Eating the placenta is called placentophagy. Placenta-ingesting enthusiasts tout its richness in iron and vitamins B6 and B12, as well as hormones such as estrogen and progesterone. In Traditional Chinese Medicine, dehydrated placenta powder is used to stimulate lactation, treat fertility disorders, and a variety of other ailments. Eating it may or may not help increase breast milk supply, boost energy levels, protect against postpartum depression, and relieve pains associated with labor and delivery. There is little scientific research on placentophagy, but many mothers attest to beneficial results. It can be washed and eaten raw, cooked like organ meat, blended into a smoothie, or made into powder and encapsulated.

A 2013 survey published in the journal *Ecology, Food, and Nutrition* is one of the few studies available on consuming the placenta. Anthropologists at the University of Las Vegas asked 189 women who ate their placentas after birth why they did it, how they preferred to have the placenta prepared, and if they would do it again. According to participants, the top three positive effects of placenta consumption were: improved mood, increased energy, and improved lactation. The top three adverse effects were: unpleasant burping, headaches, and unappealing taste or smell.

Studies have shown that consuming placenta can:
- Help to balance your hormones
- Replenish depleted iron levels
- Assist the uterus in returning to its pre-pregnancy state
- Reduce post-natal bleeding
- Increase milk production—this has been proven in a study
- Make for a happier, more enjoyable post-natal period
- Increase your energy levels

∽

Baby blues can affect up to 80% of women within the first week of birth. Women who consume their placenta report fewer emotional issues and a more enjoyable postpartum.

SOME CONTRAINDICATIONS OF INGESTING THE PLACENTA

- If the mother or newborn has a viral or bacterial infection
- If the mother has received a general anesthetic as it may have absorbed opioids and other anesthetic agents
- If the mother smoked while pregnant, that increases the concentration of cadmium in the placental tissue and thus poses a risk

PLACENTA MEDICINE

BREASTFEEDING

To understand the benefits with regard to breastfeeding, it is essential to know the process of lactation. As the placenta separates from the uterine wall during the third stage of labor, a dramatic shift in hormones takes place in the mother's brain and bloodstream. The major hormones that help during birthing, such as oxytocin and prolactin, continue to be important as breast milk production starts in the first few days after giving birth.

OXYTOCIN

Oxytocin is the hormone normally produced in the hypothalamus and released by the posterior pituitary. It plays a role in orgasm, social recognition, sexual reproduction, childbirth, and the period after delivery. In the brain, oxytocin acts as a chemical messenger and is important in human behaviors, including sexual arousal, recognition, trust, anxiety, and mother-infant bonding. This small nine amino acid peptide is involved in a wide variety of physiological and pathological functions such as sexual activity, penile erection, ejaculation, pregnancy, uterine contraction, milk ejection, maternal behavior, social bonding, stress and probably many more. As a result, oxytocin is called the 'love hormone' or 'cuddle chemical.'

In labor, oxytocin stimulates the uterine muscles to contract and increases production of prostaglandins, stimulating more contractions and more oxytocin to be released. In this way, contractions increase in intensity and frequency. When a baby sucks at the breast of its mother, the stimulation of the nipple leads to oxytocin secretion into the blood, which then causes milk to be let down into the breast. Oxytocin is released into the mother's brain to help stimulate further oxytocin secretion, which is a reason nipple stimulation is so effective in a mother's dilation process in labor.

Low oxytocin levels have been linked to autism and autistic spectrum disorders (*e.g.,* Asperger syndrome). Some scientists believe oxytocin could be used to treat these disorders.

PROLACTIN

Prolactin is the hormone that tells the body to make breast milk when a person is pregnant or breastfeeding. Production of prolactin takes place in the pituitary gland. The pituitary gland is a part of your endocrine system. It receives messages from the brain (via a gland called the hypothalamus), secretes hormones into your bloodstream, and stimulates all the other hormone-producing glands to produce their hormones. These hormones affect other organs and glands, especially the thyroid- a butterfly-shaped organ located in the base of your neck that controls metabolism—the way your body uses energy. The thyroid hormones regulate vital body functions, including heart rate, body weight, breathing, central and peripheral nervous systems, body temperature, moon cycles, and more.

The placenta has a store of oxytocin and prolactin leftover from labor. The placenta also has beneficial iron and protein to strengthen the new mother's blood and ease recovery from her birth experience, which could lead to a less fatigued mom and a better chance of bringing in a plentiful milk supply.

OTHER HORMONES

Research shows that the placenta makes many hormones and raises their levels during the end of pregnancy. The brain is usually responsible for the production of these hormones, so while the placenta is making them, the brain slows production. When the placenta is delivered, many of the hormones are still in the blood and tissues of the placenta. The hormones in the mother's bloodstream will drop dramatically at birth. The brain will take a few weeks to balance the production of the hormones, which is why many moms (as many as 80%) experience symptoms of the baby blues (emotions, mood swings, sadness). The placenta can offer an easily absorbed form of some of these hormones like estrogen, prolactin, and Corticotrophin-releasing hormone (CRH). These hormones can balance the production of serotonin, a hormone associated with feelings of happiness, help get breastfeeding off to a good start, and keep stress levels low during the postpartum period.

FATIGUE

Traditional Chinese medicine uses placenta medicine to address fatigue. Many new moms are anemic, or iron deficient. This condition sometimes occurs during pregnancy but can be brought on by blood loss during delivery. Most moms recover their iron stores due to their increased blood supply from pregnancy, but for those that are still anemic, symptoms can lead to physical fatigue, making the stress of caring for a newborn or recovering from a difficult birth even harder. Moms with fatigue that doesn't go away with rest have been shown to have a higher risk of developing postpartum depression and a lack of bonding with their newborn. The good news is that even if a mom is not iron deficient at delivery, the boost of iron from placenta medicine can raise energy levels and balance emotions by lessening the stress of the postpartum period.

PREVENTION OF POST BIRTH HEMMORAGE

from *Placenta, The Forgotten Chakra*, by Robin Lim, CPM

"When a mom begins to bleed, the midwife must be ready to use what she has on hand to reliably stop hemorrhage. For this, she may employ the placenta.

I would never have expected my friend Ingrid, a tall Dutch woman married to a man from the island of Flores, to hemorrhage after the birth of her second baby. She arrived at the airport in Bali, and her water released. She called to tell me she was beginning labor, though she thought she had three weeks more of pregnancy. I asked her to come quickly to the Bumi Sehat birth center. Almost immediately after she arrived, she was in the birth tub, and soon after, her baby girl was in her arms. "Well, I made it to Bali," Ingrid beamed at the Baliniese midwives attending her. "I was so afraid of bleeding like I did after my first baby's birth."

Unfortunately, as soon as she uttered those words, the birth tub turned a deep red. Her midwife Gung Sayang did not reach for oxytocin, as she knew from Ingrid's history that medication would not help. Instead, Gung Sayang nipped off a generous piece of the placenta, which was floating in a bowl in the birth tub, coated it with honey, and fed it to Ingrid. Ingrid was more than happy to eat placenta, as she was terrified of bleeding again. Shortly after eating a piece of her placenta, Ingrid's uterus contracted effectively, and she stopped bleeding. Her milk came in quickly, and the baby championed at feeding on her breasts. I asked Bidan Chantia, who assisted Gung Sayang that day, "Why did you give her such a big piece of the placenta to eat?" Chantia replied, "Because she is such a tall, large woman!" This brought laughter to all of us, including Ingrid, who was grateful that her baby's placenta had saved her life."

CAN BE EATEN RAW OR COOKED

There is, as mentioned above, the option to eat the placenta raw, soon after birth. I found it easy to do, as I felt invincible after birthing my son! My midwife took off a piece of my babies' placenta for me, and I washed it, chewed it up, and drank some water. The lactation consultant was impressed with how much colostrum was coming in. I told her I had eaten a piece of raw placenta, to which she replied, "Wow! Maybe that really does work!" Some people nowadays are calling the eating of the placenta cannibalistic. By definition, that would mean someone eats the flesh of another human being. This organ is not from another human being. It is grown inside a woman's body for the health and survival of her child. Interesting that eating the rotting flesh, organs, and lactation of other species such as chickens, cows, pigs, fish, deer, lambs, goats, etc. doesn't seem to be disgusting to most, but ingesting the placenta is entirely outlandish!

〰

*Placenta should be no more than 2–4 days old when prepared for ingesting. It is best if made the very day of the birth. If someone is hired to encapsulate the placenta, they will usually come to pick up from place of birth. The drying process takes about 24 hours. The next day the placenta is return, ground, put into capsules, into a jar, and placed in the fridge. If a raw placenta has been in the refrigerator for three days, and you won't be getting around to drying it, double bag it in gallon size bags and place in the freezer until you can. It can stay frozen for up to one year, but the sooner you encapsulate it, the better.

HOW TO ENCAPSULATE THE PLACENTA

To prepare the placenta according to traditional Chinese medicine:
1. Wash away excess blood.
2. Place in a steamer, shiny side down. Steam on low heat for about 15 minutes. Turn and steam 15 more minutes. (You will know it is finished if no blood comes out when you prick it with a fork.)
3. Slice placenta into thin, 1/8-inch strips.
4. Place strips in a dehydrator and dry on low heat, typically between 105–115 degrees F. This step takes 7–10 hours. Or, place strips on a cookie sheet and bake in the oven on the lowest possible setting.
5. Several hours later, when placenta strips are dehydrated, grind with a mortar and pestle. Then encapsulate the powder in vegetarian capsules.

〰

A placenta will make an average of 75–200 capsules, depending on the size of the baby, gestation, and capsule size. Take 1–2 capsules three times per day in the first couple of weeks, then 1–2 per day or as needed. The placenta powder is supposed to keep its original beneficial properties for three years if kept correctly in the fridge. An option is to dissolve the powder from the capsule in a little water during the 42 days of postpartum rest (if there is difficulty in swallowing pills).

CAN I EAT MY PLACENTA IF I CHOOSE LOTUS BIRTH?

Yes, you can. Mothers can take a small piece of the placenta immediately after birth and eat it, even if they choose not to sever the umbilical cord. This first bit of placenta food/medicine is more palatable if dipped in maple syrup or powdered cinnamon. Both taste good and enhance digestion.

CAN I STILL MAKE MY LOTUS BIRTH PLACENTA INTO MEDICINE FOR LATER USE?

Salting Lotus Birth placenta not only reduces the odor to nearly nothing, it preserves the placenta so that once the cord releases it may be used as medicine; this is accomplished by steaming the placenta, slicing it, and drying it. Next, it is pulverized and put into capsules. It may then be kept in a cool, dry place (freezer is best) and used over the course of the postpartum, or later in life to reduce symptoms of the mother's menopause.

FOR A LOTUS BIRTH

(Umbilical cord is left to fall off naturally)

1. Placenta is delivered, placed in bowl.
2. Allow all blood to go through the cord (~1 hour).
3. Take baby/placenta in bowl to sink, and wash off all excess blood from the placenta (both sides).
4. Cut a 2-inch piece of placenta from edge, using scissors or knife (tell baby it's for mom to ingest).
5. Cover placenta with rosemary powder and salt, getting into creases.
6. Place on cloth inside bamboo steamer.
7. Carry baby and placenta to bed.
8. Rosemary/salt mix should be re-applied about 2–3 times per day. Place around belly button also.
9. After cord falls off (usually 2–3 days), prepare the placenta for powder.
10. Oven-dry until like a crispy biscuit.
11. With a stone mortar and pestle grind into fine powder. A blender is easier but can transfer the sharp and speedy blender spirit into the placenta powder. The handling of it is important, since the procedure influences the result, as every cook knows! It will taste salty due to the preserving process.

COST OF ENCAPSULATION

The cost of placenta encapsulation varies between service providers. Some provide a cheaper fee if you're already a client (*e.g.,* if you've hired them as your doula or midwife). The cost can be $200–$400, depending on what is included. Options of more extensive preparations with the placenta include salves, tinctures, artwork, jewelry, etc.

DIFFERENT CULTURES AND THE PLACENTA

- In places like South Africa, Nigeria, Ghana, the native people buried it in a sacred place, and some had a particular tree under which they would plant it.
- Before the 1300's, the King of France's dried placenta preceded him on a cushion and at every procession or parade.
- Navajo tradition encourages grandmothers to bury their newborn grandchild's placenta and umbilical cord at a special place in the earth that represents their dreams for the child.
- In old Hawaii, the father of a new baby would bring the placenta to the ocean and leave it cradled in a *puka* (hole) in the volcanic stone by the sea. There the sacred organ could return home to her mother ocean.
- The Cunas, who lived in the borderlands between Columbia and Peru, believed in a placenta spirit resembling a guardian dog that helped the child navigate his soul boat on the amniotic waters through the labyrinth toward earthly life.
- To protect new mothers from infection and postpartum cramping, a Costa Rican midwife might wrap the placenta in paper and bury it in a dry hole with ashes from the cooking fire.
- In Guatemala, if the placenta is not born easily, a common remedy is to boil a purple onion in beer and have the woman drink the liquid.
- When a Mayan child is born, the placenta is buried in the ground as a ritual, symbolically "planting," the individual to root their Mayan identity. Then, the person will not become individualistic or selfish, but a part of the community, of nature and the cosmos.
- In parts of Vietnam, the placenta is buried under the mother's bed.

- In Cambodia, a spiky plant is placed over the chosen placental burial site to ward off evil spirits and dogs from what the people believe is "the globe of the origin of the soul."
- Childless women in Japan have been known to borrow the petticoat of a pregnant friend or relative and step over the burial site of a new placenta to increase fertility.
- Traditional Ukrainian midwives would look carefully at the newborn's placenta to divine just how many children this mother was destined to have. The placenta could not be buried in a doorway, or the mother would become infertile.

Several times over the years, parents have come to me repeatedly with a baby who has sniffles. When I ask, 'Where is the baby's placenta?' They answer, 'Oh it's still in the freezer. We haven't had time to give it a proper burial yet.' I advise them to get that placenta into the ground, where it will be warm and properly returned to the earth. After this, the baby's chronic colds clear completely!" – Robin Lim, midwife

"YOU DO NOT DIE ALONE"
– from *Placenta, The Forgotten Chakra,* by Robin Lim

"We are not alone in the womb. From the beginning we enjoy the comfort of our placenta twin. This sister or brother sleeps and dreams and drums with us as we develop. With our placenta we share the lullaby of our mother's heartbeat. Indeed, we are not born alone, for the placenta shares our birth with us. Due to modern birth protocols most of us are severed from this sacred twin prematurely, and we learn to fear separation, abandonment, and aloneness. If the indigenous Balinese belief has any truth to it, our placenta's body dies at birth in order to stay with us in spirit. This spirit brother or sister takes every earthly step with us. At the end of life, it helps us through the portal of death, just as it helped us navigate the portal into life, coming into the light just behind us, after guiding us through the birth canal. Once we are born, if the cord is not quickly severed, the placenta gives us her share of our blood, so that our brain, heart and all our organs are deeply enervated.

At death, our placenta appears beside us in spirit, now apparent to our 'spirit' eyes. He or she accompanies us through the tunnel of light to the other side, just as the placenta advocated for your embryonic and fetal life, so too does it testify for you in the after-life. The placenta knows our life pattern and all the promises we made before coming into incarnation. Your placenta will tell your life story, and you will see and feel and hear it all in detail, beginning from the last thing you heard in life and ending with the first word or sound you heard upon entering the world. This is why I counsel parents to whisper an intentional word or message to the baby upon birth. Imagine a world in which each new baby receives a message of love, peace, trust, and caring, to be carried by the soul. This sound, word, prayer, will take us higher when we recall, with the help of our placenta, our entire life story.

It is time we each remember and acknowledge the angel that helped us into the world and who is with us always. If you want to see the physical form of an angel, a miracle in the flesh, behold the placenta. Culture a kinship now with your placenta/guardian angel, and you may find that your life feels blessed. You may be much more at ease when facing your death. By believing in your placenta/angel, you will learn to trust the dying process as a birth process into the next phase of your soul's life. I assure you, you were not born alone, and you will not die alone."

∽

The foremost and thorough exploration and understanding of the placenta and its function comes from Ibu Robin Lim, CPM. Her book, *Placenta, The Forgotten Chakra* (Copyright 2010, Half Angel Press, Bali Indonesia), which I have cited often in this chapter, is glorious and unparalleled. Two hundred pages of content including such topics as Honoring the Third Stage of Labor: The Birth of the Placenta, Neonatal Tetanus, Burning the Cord Instructions, Cord Cutting and Disease, Rh- Mothers, Babies, and Placentas, Cord Blood Banking, How about Premature Babies? Placenta: Our Hero/

Heroine in Myth and History, Placentas and GMO Foods, Placenta Take-Home Check List, Pre-Birth Planning for Placenta Ceremony, Options for Parents to Consider when Planning Baby & Placenta's Birth, How to Keep Placenta and Placenta Ceremonies, How to Have a Lotus Birth: The Nitty-Gritty Details, Lotus Birth After Cesarean.

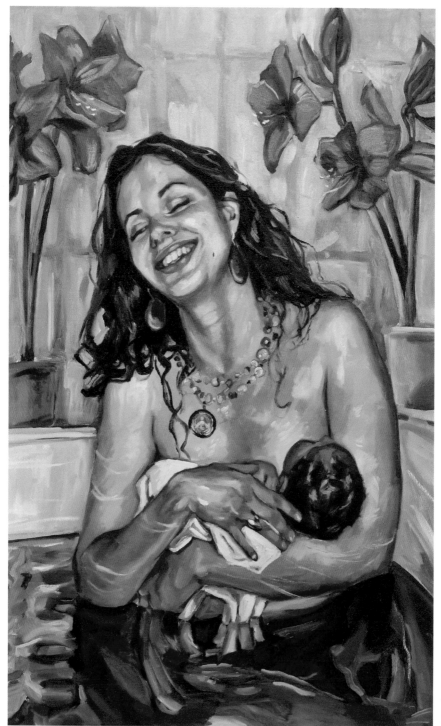

Amanda Greavette

CHAPTER 9: WATER

"There's plenty of water in the universe without life, but nowhere is there life without water."
- SYLVIA A. EARLE

"Water, thou hast no taste, no color, no odor; canst not be defined, art relished while ever mysterious. Not necessary to life, but rather life itself, thou fillest us with a gratification that exceeds the delight of the senses."
- ANTOINE DE SAINT-EXUPERY

"Water does not resist. Water flows. When you plunge your hand into it, all you feel is a caress. Water is not a solid wall, it will not stop you. But water always goes where it wants to go, and nothing in the end can stand against it. Water is patient. Dripping water wears away a stone. Remember that, my child. Remember you are half water. If you can't go through an obstacle, go around it. Water does."
- MARGARET ATWOOD
The Penelopiad

MY HUSBAND WILL TELL you if I see a body of water, I want to get in it! It is where we begin our journey in our form. It is cleansing, healing, and hydrating. Those who live in places where water is scarce and must travel to get water, rather than turn on a faucet, likely have a deeper appreciation or perhaps use it more wisely or sparingly. Our bodies are up to 60% water. According to H.H. Mitchell, Journal of Biological Chemistry 158, the brain and heart are composed of 73% water, and the lungs are about 83% water. The skin contains 64% water, muscles and kidneys are 79%, and even the bones are watery: 31%.

Water. It is the source of life. It fertilizes and impregnates the Earth, giving it life. Water is the base for all the vital fluids of the body: phlegm, mucus, plasma, lymph, kidneys, bladder and urinary tract, mucosa of the digestive, respiratory, and genitourinary tracts, the brain and spinal cord. Water is the most receptive element, the most excellent receiver and absorber of energy. It symbolizes spirit and healing. It has been used in labor for decades. Its ability to relax, warm, and nurture the birthing woman through birth is known among those who use it or who witness it. We all enter this current physical realm in the womb of our mothers and live for months in the amniotic fluid.

WHAT IS THE AMNIOTIC FLUID?
The amniotic fluid is a clear, slightly yellowish liquid that surrounds the fetus during pregnancy, and contained in the amniotic sac. While in the womb, the baby floats in the amniotic fluid. The amount of amniotic fluid is highest at about 34 weeks into the pregnancy, when it averages 800 mL. At 40 weeks, it averages about 600 mL.

Amniotic fluid is 98% water and 2% salts and cells from the baby. Until the fetal kidneys start working during month four, amniotic fluid is made by the water from the mother's body. But after month 4, the fetus begins to make its contribution to the amniotic fluid by urinating into it. The amniotic fluid continuously circulates as the baby swallows the amniotic fluid, which then passes through their digestive system, into their kidneys, and back out again to the amniotic sac as urine. So the baby is practicing urine therapy in the womb! What is urine therapy?

Urine therapy is the ingestion or topical application of one's urine and has been practiced around the world for millennia. Urine is mostly water (95%), urea (2.5%), and a mixture of uric acid, creatinine, electrolytes, phosphate and organic acids, proteins (most are albumin, which is a principal protein in breastmilk) enzymes, hormones, glucose, and water-soluble vitamins. Urine is sterile where it is produced in the kidney, but once it has left the body, it is usually contaminated, but not toxic. Only urea, the substance after which urine is named, can be poisonous when present in the blood; yet, this is irrelevant in the practice of drinking urine, as urine is not immediately put back in the bloodstream. In small amounts, urea gets back into the body, it is purifying, and clears up excess mucus. Urine is entirely sterile after secretion and has an antiseptic effect.

After the liver detoxifies blood, it flows to the kidneys. The kidneys' most crucial function is balancing out all elements in the blood. They remove all superfluous vital substances from the blood and filter out a surplus of water. This water and the vital substances consequently form urine, which is stored in the bladder until you do something with it—when you pee, or "urinate." Urine is ultra-filtered blood plasma, and may be the most nutrient-dense, mineralized drink on the planet, with anti-bacterial, anti-fungal and anti-candida properties, which are curative and strengthening. It is free, directly from yourself, and available daily, thereby not a standard recommendation for healing.

In urine therapy, the recommendation is to drink the portion from the first pee of the day, mid-flow, as it is highest in nutrients and purest. Urine might be the only option for cleaning a wound when there is a lack of pure water. People have been known to drink their urine when buried under a collapsed building after a hurricane, lost at sea for days or the original location—the womb!

By the time the baby is born, they will consume up to 15 ounces of amniotic fluid a day. At first, the fluid is mainly water with electrolytes, but around the 12–14th week, the liquid also contains proteins, carbohydrates, lipids, phospholipids, and urea, all of which aid in the growth of the fetus.

THE AMNIOTIC FLUID HELPS:

- The developing baby to move in the womb, which allows for exercising of muscles and proper bone growth.
- The lungs to develop correctly—baby breathes fluid in and out of the lungs.
- Maintain a constant temperature around the baby, protecting from heat loss.
- Cushion and protect the baby from outside injury by cushioning sudden blows or movements.
- Keep the umbilical cord from being squeezed.
- Create space for growth.
- Protect against infection—the membranes provide a barrier + the fluid contains antimicrobial peptides.
- Because the baby's body parts are growing so fast, the fluid provides lubrication that keeps them from growing together. In some cases, fingers and toes can become webbed as a result of not enough amniotic fluid circulating in the uterus.

SPONTANEOUS RUPTURE OF MEMBRANES

Around 80–90% of women start labor with their membranes intact, probably because the amniotic sac plays a vital role in the physiology of a natural birth. The forewaters are released when the amnion ruptures, which is commonly known as the time when a woman's "water breaks." When this occurs during labor at term, it is known as "spontaneous rupture of membranes." The rupture of membranes can occur at various stages of dilation. The forewaters usually break when the cervix is almost entirely open, and the membranes are bulging so far into the vagina that they burst. This 'fluid burst' lubricates the vaginal and perineum to facilitate movement of the baby and stretching of the tissues. Even after the water breaks, there is still some fluid present.

FLUID PRESSURE

Dr. Rachel Reed, in an article titled *In Defense of the Amniotic Sac*, from Midwife Thinking.com states:

> "During a contraction, the pressure is equalized throughout the fluid rather than directly squeezing the baby, placenta, and umbilical cord. This protects the baby and his/her oxygen supply from the effects of the powerful uterine contractions. When fluid is reduced (by escaping through a hole in the membranes), the placenta and baby get compressed during a contraction. Most babies can cope well with this, but the experience of birth for the baby is probably not as pleasant. When the placenta is compressed, blood circulation is interrupted, reducing the oxygen supply to the baby. In addition, the umbilical cord may be in a position where it gets squashed between baby and uterus with contractions. When this happens, the baby's heart rate will dip during a contraction in response to the reduced blood flow. A healthy baby can cope with this intermittent reduction in oxygen for hours (it's a bit like holding your breath for 30 seconds every few minutes). However, this is not optimal if for an extended period of time, especially if the baby is already compromised through prematurity or a poorly functioning placenta."

FORE WATERS & HIND WATERS

The sac of amniotic fluid is described as having two sections—the fore waters (in front of the baby's head) and the hind waters (behind baby's head). Often a hind water leak is experienced by the woman as an occasional light trickle since the fluid has to run down the outside of the sac and past the baby's head to get out.

As Dr. Reed so wonderfully explains, "During labor, fore waters are formed as the lower segment of the uterus stretches, and the chorion (the external membrane) detaches from it. The well-flexed baby's head fits into the cervix and cuts off the fluid in front of the head (fore waters) from the fluid behind (hind waters). Pressure from contractions cause the fore waters to bulge downwards into the dilating cervix and eventually through into the vagina. This protects the fore waters from the high pressure applied to the hind waters during a contraction and keeps the membranes intact. The fore waters transmit pressure evenly over the cervix, which aids dilation."

The mucous plug is an accumulation of mucous and thick fluid that seals the cervix during pregnancy, and prevents bacteria from entering the uterus. It comes out as the woman nears labor. Also called "bloody show."

THE CAUL

The amniotic membrane, a thin translucent tissue, enclosing a fetus is called the caul. If is rare for a baby to be born "en caul," occurring in about 1 in every 80,000 births. Eventually the force of the contraction and the movement of the baby will rupture the sac as the baby's body is born. Caul births are usually more common in water births. Herstorically being born in the caul was considered good luck for the baby. It was believed that a baby born in the caul would be protected from drowning. Midwives used to dry out amniotic membranes and sell them to sailors as a talisman to protect them from drowning. There are many olden day superstitions related to caul births, which can be found in Thomas R. Forbes *The Social History of the Caul*, Yale J Biol Med 1953 Jun; 25(6): 495–508).

ARTIFICIAL RUPTURE OF MEMBRANES

Artificial rupture of membranes (ARM), aka 'breaking the waters', is a common intervention during birth. However, women need to be fully informed of the risks of this intervention before agreeing to alter labor in this way. After the water breaks, usually, the mother is "on the clock" so to speak, and usually given a maximum amount of hours to birth baby before interventions are imposed.

Breaking the membranes with an amni-hook is a common intervention, usually the second step in the induction process, and done in an attempt to speed up labor. In an induced labor, intact membranes can prevent the artificially created contractions from getting into an effective pattern. There is also the theoretical risk of an induced contraction (that is too strong) forcing amniotic fluid through the membranes/placenta and into the blood system causing an amniotic embolism and maternal death. So an ARM is usually recommended before Pitocin is begun.

In a spontaneous labor, the rationale for an ARM is that once the fore-waters are gone, the hard baby's head will apply direct pressure to the cervix and open it quicker. However, a Cochrane review of the available research states, "the evidence showed no shortening of the length of first stage of labor and a possible increase in Caesarean section. Routine amniotomy is not recommended for normally progressing labors or in labors, which have become prolonged."

RISKS ASSOCIATED WITH ARTIFICAL RUPTURE OF MEMBRANES:

- Could increase intensity of contractions, which can result in the woman feeling unable to cope and opting for epidural drugs
- The baby may become distressed due to compression of the placenta, baby and/or cord
- Studies have found that amniotomy altered fetal vascular blood flow, suggesting there is a fetal stress response following an ARM
- The umbilical cord could be swept down by the waters, and either past the baby's head or wedged next to the baby's head. This is called a 'cord prolapse' and is an emergency situation. The compression of the cord interrupts or stops the supply of oxygen to the baby, and the baby must be born as soon as possible by C-section
- If there is a blood vessel running through the membranes and the amni-hook ruptures the vessel, the baby will lose blood volume fast—another emergency
- There is a slight increase in the risk of infection but mostly for the mother. This risk is minimal if nothing is put into the vagina during labor (*i.e.,* hands, instruments, etc.).

AMNIOTIC FLUID LEVELS

The standard of practice in the U.S. is to induce labor at term if a mother has low amniotic fluid in an otherwise healthy pregnancy. 95% of physicians who practice maternal-fetal medicine feel that isolated oligohydramnios—low amniotic fluid in an otherwise healthy pregnancy—is an indication for labor induction at 40 weeks. (J Matern Fetal Neonatal Med, April 22, 2009, "Practice patterns in the management of isolated oligohydramnios: a survey of perinatologists," Schwartz, Sweeting, Young BK)

Because the mother's fluid levels are the source of amniotic fluid, changes in the mother's fluid status can result in changes in the amount of amniotic fluid. Amniotic fluid levels increase until the mother reaches about 34–36 weeks, and then levels gradually decline until birth. The baby will swallow more fluid towards the end of term, which will lead to lower levels. If a mother is dehydrated, this will lower the levels. If the baby has a congenital disability, or a kidney or urinary tract issue, the levels could be lower. If the mother has preeclampsia or intrauterine growth restriction, the levels may be lower.

It is important to understand that amniotic fluid levels exist on a continuum and that there is no agreement among researchers about the cut-off value that predicts poor outcomes.

To read more on how amniotic fluid is measured, accuracy, evidence and results of studies, visit Lamaze.org and EvidenceBasedBirth.com.

WHAT IS MECONIUM?

The baby's first stool, or feces, is called meconium. It is a dark greenish substance, sticky, and thick in nature. Most babies poop for the first time outside of the womb, but 6–25% of newborns have meconium-stained amniotic fluid, which means they had the bowel movement before birth. After 40 weeks gestation around 20% of babies will pass meconium into their amniotic fluid as the bowels reach maturity and begin to work. This is perfectly normal and not a guaranteed sign of distress. This meconium is diluted and processed with the amniotic fluid. Of the 6–25% of newborns who poop in utero, only about 11% of them will have *some degree* of Meconium Aspiration Syndrome (MAS). Severe and rare cases of MAS, occurring in 0.04% of all births, lead to lung collapse, aspiration pneumonia, or lung disease.

MAS can occur when the baby inhales a mixture of meconium and amniotic fluid. The inhaled meconium can partially or completely block the baby's airways. Although air can flow past meconium as the baby inhales, the meconium becomes trapped in the airways when the baby exhales, irritating the airways and making it difficult to breathe. MAS can happen before, during, or after labor and delivery.

Current guidelines state that if a newborn has inhaled meconium but looks well, is crying, active, and has a strong heartbeat and no fetal distress (>100 bpm), the delivery team can watch the baby for MAS symptoms (such as increased respiratory rate, grunting, or cyanosis), which usually appear in the first 24 hours. There would be no suctioning or intervention, and baby can be given to the mother for immediate skin-to-skin, while APGAR scores are done by the care provider. If the newborn has inhaled meconium and is limp, a low heart rate (<100bpm), poor muscle tone, and not very active, the protocol is to clear the airway to decrease the amount of meconium the baby inhales.

If a mother's water breaks and there is meconium in the fluid, there will be a greenish tint or streaks. This should be communicated to the care provider if they are not in the room. If at a hospital setting, the mother would then be given a fetal monitor to check for any signs of distress. If in a homebirth, midwives do carry tools to help suction meconium and normal secretions, but the midwife may opt for a transport to the hospital.

GOOD TO KNOW...

Water acts as a transport system to carry nutrients through the blood to you and the baby.

- Dehydration can cause contractions, and lack of water in the third trimester can also cause premature labor.
- The more water you drink during pregnancy, the less water your body will retain.
- Not drinking enough water can lead to constipation, headaches, nausea (and other morning sickness symptoms), and fatigue.
- Staying well hydrated is also a great way to reduce the chances of stretch marks.
- Water flushes out the system. Increasing water intake will dilute the urine and help prevent urinary tract infections, which are common in pregnancy (and uncomfortable).

When a woman in labor relaxes in a warm deep bath, free from gravity's pull on her body with sensory stimulation reduced, her body is less likely to secrete stress-related hormones. This allows her body to produce the pain inhibitors—endorphins—that complement labor. A laboring woman who is able to relax physically is able to relax mentally as well.

BENEFITS OF HYDROTHERAPY DURING LABOR & BIRTHING

Benefits of water labor and water birth, highly rated by both mothers and experienced providers, and which research has verified, are as follows:

- The effect of buoyancy that water immersion creates allows spontaneous movement of the mother. Water facilitates mobility and enables the mother to assume any position, which is comfortable for labor and birth. Movement helps open the pelvis, allowing the baby to descend
- Speeds up labor
- Reduces blood pressure
- Gives mother more feelings of control
- Provides significant pain relief
- Promotes relaxation
- Conserves her energy
- Reduces the need for drugs and interventions
- Gives mother a private protected space
- Reduces perineal trauma and eliminates episiotomies
- Reduces cesarean section rates
- Encourages an easier birth for mother and a gentler welcome for baby. Placing a pool of water in a birth room changes the atmosphere immediately. Voices get softer, the mother stays calmer, and everyone becomes less stressed

ABOUT BARBARA HARPER OF WATERBIRTH INTERNATIONAL

Barbara Harper, founder of Waterbirth International, promotes water birth around the world, striving to make it an available option for all women. Her expertise is sought in all areas of the globe. She has lectured in 43 countries, including medical schools, nursing schools, midwifery programs, and university women's studies departments. She has been interviewed by hundreds of newspapers and magazines and appeared on dozens of radio and TV shows to talk about her work.

Barbara started her career in maternity as a registered nurse, and was always passionate about mothers and babies, even in nursing school. Her maternal grandmother was a nurse and midwife for 47 years. She founded Waterbirth International in 1987 after visiting Russia for the first time and sitting down with Igor Charkovsky, who's complete faith in birthing women and their babies influenced her. She worked extensively with Binnie Dansby in the early 1980's, learning to respect the cognitive, but repressed, experiences and memories of birth in all our lives.

Her research and experiences resulted in the publication of *Gentle Birth Choices*, a book and DVD, and all-time best-seller in childbirth books. Midwives and parents alike have called her video programs, "the most inspiring birth videos ever produced." The following information is from her website waterbirth.org:

Where can one purchase a birth pool?
We recommend waterbirthsolutions.com for all waterbirth pools and supplies for parents, waterbirth professionals and institutions.

How long does it take to blow up the tub?
Birth pools are designed for set up in less than 20 minutes, though the filling may take an hour or so. Mother or partner may wish to practice setting up the tub a few times if they will be the one to set up at labor.

What is the temperature of the water?
Water should be maintained and monitored at a temperature that is comfortable for the mother, usually between 92–100 degrees Fahrenheit (32–38 degrees Celsius).

When should the mother get into the water?
A woman should be encouraged to use the labor pool whenever she wants. Some mothers find a bath in early labor useful for its

calming effect and to determine if labor has started. If contractions are strong and regular, no matter how dilated the cervix is, a bath might help the mother relax enough to facilitate dilation. It has been suggested that the tub be used as a "trial of water" for at least one hour to allow the mother to judge its effectiveness. Midwives report that some women can go from 1 cm to complete dilation within the first hour or two of immersion. Research studies have demonstrated that water is an effective tool to assist irregular contractions in becoming more consistent or in using water immersion instead of Pitocin for a stalled labor. This reaction is due to an increase in Oxytocin levels and a reduction of stress hormones.

How long is baby in the water after they arrive?
Babies should be gently lifted out of the water without hurrying or rushing. Anyone can do this, including the mother herself. It is beneficial for the provider to allow the baby to emerge entirely in the water, examine for cord entanglement, and unwind the cord before lifting the baby out of the water. All accomplished in a few seconds. Remind the mother to raise the baby slowly if she is the one reaching down because you don't know how long the cord is. Research studies indicate that there are more cord ruptures or breaking of the cord, caused by quickly jerking the baby out of the water.

Remember that physiologically, the placenta is still supporting the baby with oxygen throughout the birth and immediately afterward. It can not be predicted when the placenta will begin to separate, causing the flow of oxygen to stop. The umbilical cord pulsating is not a guarantee that the baby is receiving enough oxygen. The safe approach is to remove the baby, without hurrying, and gently place him upright onto the mother's chest or hold the baby, suspended with the head out of the water, until the mother reaches down to lift the baby up.

Reasons a woman may not be able to birth in water:

If the baby is in breech position, if the mother has been diagnosed with excessive bleeding or maternal infection, if she is having multiples, or if preterm labor is expected. Discussing with healthcare provider whether she is a candidate for a water birth is essential.

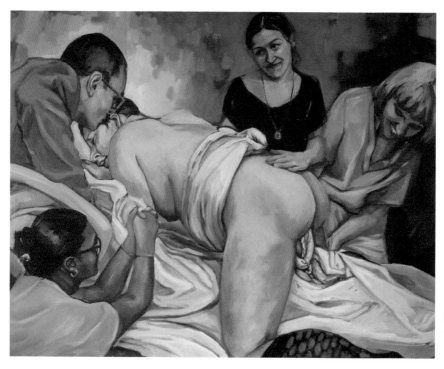

Amanda Greavette

CHAPTER 10:
LABOR & BIRTH

"It is said that women in labor leave their bodies...
they travel to the stars to collect the souls of their
babies and return to this world together."
- ANONYMOUS

"It is not only that we want to bring about an easy labor,
without risking injury to the mother or the child; we must go
further. We must understand that childbirth is fundamentally
a spiritual, as well as a physical, achievement... The birth
of a child is the ultimate perfection of human love."
- DR. GRANTLY DICK-READ, 1953

"Remember that each labor contraction is caused by a wave of
Oxytocin (the love hormone) coursing through your body. So, very
literally, each birthing surge is a surge of love. Allow yourself to
meet each surge with the same warmth, intimacy and acceptance
that you would experience during a kiss or a loving embrace."
- LAURALYN CURTIS

LABOR WILL PRESENT ITSELF differently to every mom, for each birth. It can start and stop, go swiftly or slowly. Labor can bring forth a determination and surrender if the woman is willing to let go of her preconceived notions of who she is. The surges that come into the body to bring the baby out are not stronger or bigger than she because they are her. My primary focus in labor was to trust, allow it to unfold without trying to control it, and connect to myself, baby, and the source for who we are: infinite, intelligent, unlimited. Labor is the work/joy of birthing. No one knows the exact mechanism that starts labor. Ancient texts suggest that the baby meditates on the mother, like knocking on a door exclaiming, "Mom, I'm ready now!"

"Through the months, mother has inwardly prepared for a very particular play, yet when performance time comes, she must throw out all scripts and trust herself to do that which she is guided to do in each moment. Patience, loving presence, support, and suggestions are all mother needs in her dance towards empowerment…No matter how it presents itself, your labor is perfect. Labor can look many ways with all sorts of time frames and still be perfect. Birth takes trust. Trust that the baby's soul is a vast Intelligence that leads you in the birthing dance, in perfect timing. Trust in the baby's script, designed by the baby's soul, and relax into whatever is happening. Trust that the mother's body does indeed know how to give birth." – Sunni Karll, Sacred Birthing

STAGES OF LABOR

FIRST STAGE:

During the first stage of labor, contractions cause the cervix to thin (effacement) and open (dilation). Thinning is given in percentage (100% effaced) and opening in centimeters (10cm dilated).

Early labor: the cervix opens to 4 centimeters. The mother can keep doing usual activities. Relax, rest, drink clear fluids, and eat light meals or snacks if desired. Contractions may slow down or go away, but eventually they'll become stronger. When they become more frequent, longer, and stronger, active labor is likely beginning.

Active labor: the cervix opens from 4 to 7 centimeters. Contractions are every 3 to 4 minutes, last about 60 seconds, and are intense for about 2 hours straight. For second time moms, contractions are every five minutes for an hour. The mother may no longer talk and will become more internal. The water may break, and contractions will then speed up.

Transition to second stage: the cervix opens from 7 to 10 centimeters. Contractions last about 60 to 90 seconds and come every 2 to 3 minutes. There is less time to rest in between. The mother may be tired, sweaty, shaky, hot and/or cold, nauseous, feeling the need to poop, opposition to touch, feeling a lot of sensation in the lower back, as well as the cervix. Sometimes she will begin lifting her heels off the floor due to the pressure she feels from the baby's head, buttocks, or feet.

Midwives recommend, when labor begins, in the first stage, to walk around, move, and do regular life things until that stage comes to a close. Staying upright quickens labor by 36% for first babies and 25% for others.

SECOND STAGE:

The second stage of labor is from full dilation of the cervix to the birth of the baby. The baby moves down the birth canal and there will be natural surges that cue the mother as to when to bear down. Meeting these surges of pressure when they arrive, will continue to bring the baby down and out. Let the uterus do the work. A mother may be vocal during this stage, groaning or grunting to help her bring the baby forth.

When the baby's head crowns, some mothers experience a burning sensation, often referred to as "the ring of fire," as the baby stretches the vaginal opening. Going slow and breathing deep can reduce the chance of tearing.

THIRD STAGE:

After the birth of the baby, the placenta detaches from the uterine wall, as the uterus continues contracting. Birthing the placenta feels like a blob, since it does not have bones like the baby. Usually, the placenta is born about 5–20 minutes after the baby. The cord does not need to be tugged on.

FOURTH STAGE:

Both baby and placenta have been born, and the mother is likely feeling fatigue. Breastfeeding as soon as possible helps the uterus contract and decrease the amount of bleeding. The care provider will press on the uterus to check if it is firming up.

LABOR POSITIONS

Most often, television, film, and the media portray a woman lying on her back, knees up, yelling. Lying on the back is not the only option for labor and may not be the most conducive. It puts more weight on the tailbone, which can be more painful for the mother. In upright positioning, there is less risk of compressing the mother's aorta, which means better oxygen supply to the baby. Also, the uterus contracts more efficiently, helping the baby get in a better position to pass through the pelvis. The principles of physics apply to childbirth. Gravity works! Most ancient sculptures show a woman crouching down, in a squat or something of that nature, to give birth. Moving the pelvis helps the baby navigate their way down.

HANDS & KNEES/KNEELING
On one knee or two (this is especially helpful if the baby's shoulders are stuck). The mother can lean on a birth ball (exercise ball) for support.

SQUATTING
Helps baby descend into the canal. It can improve the quality of contractions while relieving pressure in the lower back and can shorten the pushing phase. Squatting opens up the pelvis. Can be done on a bed, floor, or birth stool, using a squat bar, birthing ball, or a person for support. Take breaks in between squats with another position.

FACING STURDY OBJECTS
Face a chair or other piece of furniture, hospital bed, bar at the end of the bed, etc. Lean on it with arms draped over or hold onto it. If in a water tub, lean against the side of it.

STANDING
Stand while wrapping arms around partner or doula's neck. Or place hands onto a wall for support.

LUNGING
Place one foot up on a bed or chair and bending the knee.

BIRTHING CHAIR
A seat that has been around for millennia, that is shaped to assist a woman in the physiological upright posture during birthing, providing balance and support. If backless, it is known as a birth stool. Often the arms will have

armrests or handholds for the mother to grip, providing extra leverage. They are traced back to Egypt in 1450 B.C.E (photos of queens birthing on stools), Greece in 200 B.C (featured on ancient sculptures), and Celtic items from 100 B.C.E. The birthing chair/stool began to resurface more around the 1980's.

SITTING ON A TOILET
Sit on a toilet facing backward, place a pillow or towel to lean on, or rest the head. This will aid in relaxing the sphincter muscles since we associate a toilet with letting go in that area.

SIDE LYING
This is helpful if mother is tired. Placing a pillow or peanut ball in between thighs is good.

DRINKS FOODS/HERBS FOR LABORING

YOUNG COCONUT WATER
Direct from the coconut is full of electrolytes, fiber, vitamin C, and an excellent source of hydration, as it is 94% water. If not available, boxed coconut water is also excellent. Potassium helps keep fluid and electrolyte balance in the body, especially during physical exertion. Because there is more potassium than sodium in coconut water, the potassium may help balance out sodium's effect on blood pressure and possibly even lower it. Electrolytes are minerals that help maintain proper fluid balance and include potassium, magnesium, sodium, and calcium. Coconut water keeps mother hydrated while providing a little boost when necessary.

WARM VEGETABLE BROTH
This can be grounding and give some energy.

DILUTED FRESH VEGETABLE JUICE
For nutrients. Add some apple for a little sugar.

WATER
Purified water with electrolytes or vitamin C will keep mother hydrated.

BASICS FOR LABORING

- Stay well hydrated. Electrolytes are also good. Dehydration is related to fatigue, which may impact the mother's tolerance and physical capacity. Staying hydrated will keep energy up, and help labor to progress. Liquids during labor: 4 ounces per hour.
- Rest when you need to.
- Empty the bladder at least once per hour.
- Receive gentle massage with warm sesame oil between contractions, focusing on the waist, sides, back, and thighs.
- Lubrication with olive oil or wheat germ oil on the mother's perineum can help ease delivery.
- Get primal! Deep guttural open-jaw sounds help pelvic floor to release.
- Blow through the lips. A loose mouth makes a loose bottom.
- Walking/moving/swiveling hips between contractions can help labor to progress.
- Deep breathing and spontaneous singing supports the downward flow of energy needed for delivery.
- Nourishment! Ayurveda advises room temperature or warm food and drink, such as a warm, nourishing broth, to provide steadiness and strength. Ice can break the mind/body-belly coordinated consciousness; however, some moms use ice to crunch on or keep cool when body temperature rises.
- Quiet and low light in the room supports mother's needed inward attention to the natural processes and signals of labor and birth and reduces stimulation of the cerebral cortex (thinking part of the brain).

"We were actually making our own culture about birth in which fear was not going to be a big part. If a woman is afraid she won't be relaxed. So you kind of go, what's going to work with her? Am I going to help her relax physically? Am I going to help her relax by showing her a technique of breathing more slowly and deeply? Which is a big one. Or am I just going to help her laugh? In one case I realized that I was just dealing with a woman whose baby was coming fast and she needed to relax fast or she was going to get a big tear and have a lot of pain. I thought, hey she is a singer. If I got her to sing she would relax.

That was just an idea that occurred to me and I grabbed it and it worked." – Ina May Gaskin, Midwife, Founder of The Farm

THINGS TO COMMUNICATE TO YOUR PARTNER BEFORE THE LABOR AND BIRTH:

- Support me with your love and trust
- Have faith in me and my innate wisdom as well as my body's and the baby's
- Do not be a cheerleader
- Let go of all your fear
- You are my advocate
- Don't take what I do in labor personally (*e.g.,* I ask you not to touch me, yell, etc.)
- Stay hydrated and eat something small if need be to keep up your energy

WHAT IF LABOR IS STALLED?
– an excerpt from a workshop with midwife Ina May Gaskin

"I would suggest that that time limit be taken away, especially if the baby is crowning. If you can see the color of the baby's skin, and it is not sheet white, there is nothing to worry about. I think that you probably have fewer tears if the mother was on her hands and knees, so I would like to see a lot of them on hands and knees while pushing. You don't want her to take a breath and hold it and push. I like to let the uterus do the work, and I don't tell her push. Just let it come. Learn to relax when you see the baby's head in view, and make it a lot of deep breathing. Slow deep breathing. When you see the elephant give birth, the elephant puts her trunk back over her head. As this big thing is coming out of her bottom, she is going 'Ahhh.' Wide as the mouth can go. I think that helps. I don't think that each woman is made different from anybody else. I think it's a matter of let's get enough calm into the birth room so we don't have a problem so much. We don't have the clock ticking away. Or somebody saying 'Hurry, hurry.'"

THINGS TO PACK IN YOUR BAG (if not birthing at home)

- birth plan
- warm clothing
- pajamas
- warm socks and slippers
- energy bars
- easily digestible snacks like fruit
- thermos with filtered water
- stainless steel straw
- speakers for music
- electronic candles
- essential oils
- visuals (affirmation cards to hang, photo, etc.)
- scarf to cover the clock
- witch hazel to dilute and put in peri bottle for after toilet use
- non-toxic pads for underwear
- blanket for baby
- clothes for baby
- pillow, blanket, & hand towel (if you prefer more softness)

THE "I'M GONNA GET HUGE" STORY
– an excerpt from a workshop with midwife Ina May Gaskin

"One time a mother was going to have a breech baby, and the bottom of the baby came first, the legs and feet were up by the face. So this is quite a big thing, and before it was really pushing her open, she was already open. It looked like an Amish woman having baby number seven or eight. I thought this is number one, what's going on?

Then I asked her later, 'How did you do that?'

And she said, 'Well, I used the mantra you gave me.'

I said, 'I didn't know I gave you a mantra.'

She said, 'When I told you how afraid I was that maybe the baby's head would get caught, you said no, you are going to get huge, and you showed me with your hands.'

Every time she pushed, it was kind of a long pushing phase, maybe 5 hours, and we don't always have a five-hour push with a breech and when we do we listen after every push with the Doppler, and the baby's heart was great. So she was already well open. Every time she pushed, she thought, "I am going to get huge, I am going to get huge. That was her mantra."

NATURAL RELIEF FOR LABOR SENSATIONS

1. MASSAGE

Touch releases oxytocin, the love hormone, relieving stress, and fear. It helps turn off the pain receptors so one doesn't feel as much pain as she would have without it.

2. AROMATHERAPY

Essential oils have been used during labor for centuries and are proven to help relax the mother, relieve stress, act as a uterine tonic, stimulate circulation, and much more. Use with a carrier oil, such as coconut, jojoba, or sweet almond oil.

BENEFICIAL OILS FOR LABOR:

Lavender: One of the most popular used in labor. Helps with relaxation and promotes calm. Also, a painkiller that stimulates circulation and healing, and may strengthen contractions.

Clary Sage: Use to strengthen contractions. Avoid during pregnancy before the baby's due date. Also reduces anxiety.

Geranium: Helps breathing and boosts circulation.

Peppermint: Helps with nausea and headaches.

Chamomile: Soothing and calming, helps reduce tensions and anxiety.

Neroli: Calming, reassuring, relaxing, and a powerful anti-depressant.

Bergamot: Uplifts and refreshes.

Jasmine: Acts as a painkiller and is known to strengthen contractions. Can be used in a compress to aid delivery of the placenta.

Marjoram: Aids breathing, helps lower blood pressure and is a pain reliever.

Ylang-Ylang: Encourages relaxation and lowers blood pressure.

Frankincense: Can be rubbed onto perineum to prevent tearing, as it promotes skin elasticity. It can ease back pain.

3. COLD & HOT COMPRESSES

Both cold and hot can be used to reduce pain and increase comfort during labor and childbirth.

COLD:

- A cold washcloth on the face, neck, and upper chest helps refresh and relax the laboring mom.
- If the mother experiences nausea, a cold washcloth on the back of the neck can help.
- A cold pack on the lower back can help with back labor or back pain.
- Ice packs on the perineum immediately after birth helps reduce swelling.

HOT:

- Warm, wet towels, a hot pack, a hot water bottle, or heating pad placed below the belly provides comfort in labor.
- Right before pushing, place a warm, wet washcloth on the perineum to reduce perineal discomfort and encourage softening and stretching of the perineal tissues in preparation for birth.
- A hot water bottle or hot pack on the back can ease back pain during labor.
- After birth, during breastfeeding, it helps to have a warm pack or a heating pad on the belly to help alleviate the cramping sensation as the uterus shrinks back to its original size.

4. HYDROTHERAPY

The use of water for physical or psychological benefits is something that many women enjoy during labor. It is more difficult to remain tense in water. Benefits of being in water (shower, tub, creek, pool):

- Ease of movement with greater mobility due to buoyancy
- Relaxation during and between contractions
- Safe and effective pain management
- Reduction of blood pressure
- A sense of control as the mother occupies her warm, private space
- Can help with cervical dilation

5. MUSIC

Music is a beautiful tool for distraction, giving the mother something to hear/focus on rather than contractions. It can bring about a feeling of ease and provide another sacred element to the atmosphere.

6. FOCUSED BREATHING

Breathing brings focus and purpose to each contraction, making contractions more productive. The mother remains relaxed and will respond more positively to what she is feeling. The steady rhythm of breathing provides a sense of wellbeing and control. Increased oxygen provides strength and energy for both the mother and baby.

7. COUNTER PRESSURE & SQUEEZING THE HIPS

Counter pressure is something that the majority of laboring women enjoy since it relieves back labor and other area-specific discomfort. Have a support person apply heavy pressure on the lower back or space that is feeling the contraction, with the entire palm of their hand. Or place hands on the lower hips, pressing in towards the center. This double hip squeeze encourages baby to descend, rotate if need be, stabilizes the sacrum, and alleviates pain.

8. ACCUPRESSURE

Acupressure is simple and can be used to relieve pain and increase contractions, among other things. It's non-invasive and does not produce any of the undesirable or potentially harmful side effects that pharmacological pain relief can. By applying pressure on specific points with your fingers, elbows, palms, or blunt-tipped instruments, you can relieve discomfort, help babies descend and engage, dilate the mother's cervix, induce labor, and strengthen contractions (especially in slow, non-progressive labors). It can also be used to alleviate nausea, combat fatigue in protracted labor, and assist posterior positioned babies to turn to an optimal anterior position for a more comfortable birth.

9. FOCAL POINT

If contractions are intense, just looking at something and focusing on it—a crack in the wall, a button on the support person's shirt, or a photograph, can help. The brain processes the information you're seeing—leaving less brain activity to process the pain you are experiencing, so you'll feel less of it. Non-painful input closes the nerve "gates" to painful input, preventing pain sensation from traveling to the central nervous system; this is called the Gate Control Theory.

10. VISUALIZATION

When you close your eyes and envision a relaxing place—a sunny beach, a blue sky, or a pristine lake, you transport your mind there. Laboring moms can visualize their cervix opening, the baby descending into the birth canal, or the breath as it enters and exits their body.

11. POSITION CHANGES

Different positions can aid the progress of labor and reduce pain sensations by increasing the pelvic opening. Staying in one position for too long can stall the labor progress and make the contractions more painful over time. So make sure to change position every 30 minutes or at the longest every hour. Someone on the birthing team can help with this.

12. VOCALIZATION

When we experience pain or discomfort, it's reasonable to use our voices to help with the pain. For example, we all make noises when we stub our toe. Vocalization is a powerful tool. A birthing woman may choose to moan, softly sing, chant, or grunt. She needs to follow her body and know that making sounds is good, it's natural, and it helps. No apologies necessary.

13. HYPNOTHERAPY

During pregnancy, through classes, videos, and audiotapes, women can learn a conditioned reflex to create a state of concentration, become deeply relaxed, and free of fear, so the uterine muscles can work with minimal pain.

14. BIRTH DOULA

Women not only need information to have a better birthing experience, but they also need physical and emotional support. Studies have shown that women supported by other women experience more positive, less complicated births and report more satisfaction with their birth experiences. They also show less use of interventions during birthing and quicker recoveries.

15. DIMMED LIGHTS

The majority of women go into labor in the middle of the night, which is no accident. Our melatonin levels increase at night and allow our bodies to relax and begin labor. When mothers are exposed to light in labor, it has been shown to slow contractions, or even stop them altogether. A cozy, comfortable, dark or dimly lit space facilitates an effective labor with lower levels of stress hormones, allowing a woman to access the part of her primitive brain that sets up the process of hormonal ebb and flow, providing the smoothest functioning of the birth process. We share this need for privacy during labor with virtually all other female mammals.

16. SEXUALITY

Ignoring the sexual aspect of labor and birth can work against progress in labor. Sexual energy can make labor more effective and less painful without medication. Specifically, nipple stimulation can help with dilation, moving labor along, relaxing the mother. Also, masturbation and kissing can do the same.

17. BIRTH BALL AND/OR PEANUT BALL

A birth ball is an exercise ball. It comforts and strengthens the lower back when sitting on it. The pelvis is also better supported and symmetrical, which provides more comfort to a laboring mother.

A peanut ball is a therapy ball shaped like a peanut and placed between the legs when lying on the side. Women can become tired in labor and sometimes need to sit down or lie down. A birth ball or a peanut ball can help them do just that, but remain comfortable and help the labor progress.

18. EAT AND DRINK

For years, women have not been allowed to eat or drink fluids during labor. Some hospitals are continuing this today. But a new study by the American Society of Anesthesiologists suggests that this may not be a good thing. The research shows most healthy women would benefit from a light meal during labor. They concluded that moms in labor need the same kind of energy and calories as marathon runners. You are working so hard, and you need the fuel to continue and remain hardy and comfortable. When you don't have that fuel, it can reduce your contractions, which then leads to a more prolonged labor. So have light snacks and fluids to keep your energy up.

19. USE THE RESTROOM

Emptying the bladder will feel more comfortable, and allow better progression. It will also ensure the bladder is not holding the baby's head up from pressing on the cervix (which aids dilation). Pooping is great, as it clears everything out and makes room for the fetus to come down. Sitting on a toilet and relaxing the anus can move things along.

20. WALK OR MOVE

It's incredibly uncomfortable for a laboring woman to remain still while experiencing real labor contractions. The more a mother moves around and is upright during labor, the more the baby is encouraged to descend into the birth canal.

21. ARM WRESTLING!

Contracting the arm muscles during labor distracts a woman's attention from holding their pelvic and thigh muscles tight to "protect themselves" during labor.

22. FOCUS ON THE 3RD EYE

Located between the eyebrows, it corresponds directly to the pituitary gland, which releases oxytocin. Oxytocin, in turn, makes the uterus contract. Your brain is continually regulating labor as it takes in many different messages, including clues about your emotional state. Fear and anxiety shut down the flow of oxytocin, can make labor more difficult, and even stop it. Closing the eyes and gazing at the point between the eyebrows is incredibly useful.

23. CHUNG & SHAKING THE APPLES

Use a technique of shaking the mother's bottom up and down or her thighs from side to side (German people call this "shaking the apples"). In China, when a woman has a long and difficult labor, to help her loosen, midwives will "chung" the mother. Chung means that 2 or 3 women shake the laboring woman vigorously all over her body, while the woman is standing, leaning over something, with her arms braced.

24. LAUGHTER

Laughing helps open up the sphincters! A good belly laugh is one of the most effective forms of anesthesia.

25. ATMOSPHERE

Anyone fearful, negative, pushy, or disrespectful, ask them to leave the room. Keep the room sacred and full of love and positivity. Keep televisions off and mundane conversations out of the room/house.

26. CHOOSING WHO YOU WANT THERE AT BIRTH

Who will be positive, supportive, and of service? Are you comfortable with them? Will they stress you in any way? Are there too many people? Do you want your children there (if not first birth)?

27. MANTRA

Mantra is a Sanskrit word comprised of of 'man-,' the mind and 'tra-,' to protect. Mantra is the repetition of an elevated phrase or word that will help protect the true nature of the mind, which is spaciousness, consciousness, and infinite. Mantra protects the mind from negativity and overwhelming thoughts.

28. DANCE, HUG, KISS, LET GO

Playfulness and intimacy can go a long way. What got the baby in can get the baby out! No need to be self conscious about making noises or pooping during labor. Get into whatever position feels best!

> "In labor, call upon something bigger than you. Call upon all the souls of the women before you in all time to help bring your baby forth into this world. Realize the infinity in the collective strength of women. Lose all thought. Ride each wave and let it go. Be present to what is happening. The biggest word is surrender. Lean on the creator to bring the baby out, as you are not the one ultimately, who made the baby. The power belongs to the one who created the stars from dust. Yet you are not separate from that power. Patience pays." – Gurumukh Kaur Khalsa, *Bountiful, Beautiful, Blissful*

∽

"What if we referred to the sensations of labor with a word other than "PAIN"? The word PAIN is so small and limited. When I stub my toe, I feel pain. When I eat something that gives me gas, I feel pain. I wish I had a better word to describe what it actually FELT like to birth my babies. There was definitely sensation. A LOT of sensation. I could feel it. But it was good. It was OK! I even enjoyed it. It was so primal and sensual...I guess you could say the pain of childbirth felt really...good. I wish I could invent a new word for it. The closest word I can think of is POWER, but mixed with surrender, sensuality, sexuality, vulnerability and strength. We belittle women and the birth experience when we refer to it with the same word we use for broken bones and bruises. The pain of labor is transcendent."
– Lauralyn Curtis, HBCE

COMMON NEWBORN PROCEDURES TO LEARN ABOUT

1. **Cord Clamping and Cutting:** See Umbilical Cord chapter.
2. **Routine Bulb Suctioning:** Can be reserved for infants who actually need it.
3. **Weighing & Measuring:** There is an obsession with what the baby weighs and measures. It is good to remember that babies are just as tall 6 hours hours after birth as they are a few minutes after birth. It can wait. So bonding is prioritized and motherbaby are not separated.
4. **Swaddling/Wrapping with Blanket:** Skin-to-skin is best for both mother and baby. Place a blanket on top of the baby once the baby is atop the mother.
5. **Baby Hat:** Being with mother skin to skin will generate the most warmth. Adjust the temperature in the room to make it less cold. Then mother can smell and see and feel the baby's head fully.
6. **PKU heel prick:** Blood is taken from a prick in the heel usually at least 24 hours after birth, to test for a rare condition called phenylketonuria (PKU), which can harm a baby's growing brain.

7. **Erythromycin Eye Ointment:** Newborns receive this to prevent pink eye in the first month of life, also called ophthalmia neonatorum (ON). The most common cause of ON is chlamydia, a sexually transmitted infection. If you tested negative for STDs in the first trimester and are in a monogamous relationship, odds are you can skip this.

8. **Vitamin K:** Newborns routinely receive an injection in the upper thigh within the first 6 hours to prevent vitamin K deficiency bleeding. Some moms opt to give an oral version called Bio-K-Mulsion or take a supplement to increase levels in breastmilk. If choosing the shot, wait several hours, ask for a preservative-free version, and comfort baby while administered. Investigate more at EvidenceBasedBirth.com.

9. **Bath:** See Vernix chapter.

10. **Hepatitis B vaccine:** Hepatitis B is transmissible when blood, semen, or another bodily fluid from a person with the virus enters the body of an individual who does not have it. Infection of the virus can occur when a mother with HBV gives birth, during sexual activity, sharing needles and syringes, unsafe tattoo techniques, and sharing of personal hygiene items. Common side effects include: discomfort around the injection site for hours or days after getting the shot, headache, nausea, vomiting, diarrhea, high temperature, fatigue, irritability, stomach pain. Rare side effects include: joint pain, pins and needles, swelling, hives, rashes, low blood pressure, and hypotension. The "Hep B" vaccine was first recommended for all infants at birth back in 1991. The injection is genetically engineered recombinant viral DNA inserted into a yeast cell. In 2017, the American Academy of Pediatrics updated their statement to suggest infants receive their first dose of the three- or four-dose hepatitis B vaccine within 24 hours of birth if they're medically stable and weigh at least four pounds, six ounces. Investigate more at KellyBroganMD.com

11. **Newborn Hearing Screening Test:** Used to examine the baby's hearing. Sounds are played and responses measured using either the Otoacoustic Emissions test or the Auditory Brainstem Response test (or both). The test takes about five to ten minutes, is and is suggested

to have done before one month old. Hospitals, clinics, and some birth centers and pediatrician offices will offer the screening.

12. **Bilirubin Test:** A diagnostic blood test to measure the levels of bilirubin (a yellow-orange bile pigment) in blood serum and to help evaluate liver function. Immediately after birth, more bilirubin is produced than the infant's immature liver can handle, and the excess remains circulating in the blood. This situation results in jaundice in over 60 percent of newborns. The jaundice usually resolves on its' own within a few weeks. The baby nursing helps the bilirubin passes through their body. Most pediatricians perform bilirubin tests every 4-6 hours in the first 24 hours after birth to monitor the levels. Normal indirect bilirubin would be under 5.2 mg/dL within the first 24 hours, but many newborns have some kind of jaundice and bilirubin levels that are between 5 and 10mg/dL. Since 97% of term babies have serum bilirubin values <13 mg/dl, all infants with a serum bilirubin level >13 mg/dl will require a minimum treatment. Severely high levels can lead to hyperbilirubinemia, which can lead to cerebral palsy, deafness and brain damage (kernicterus). The treatment for abnormally high levels is phototherapy, where the baby wears eye covers and is placed under "Bili lights" and/or given a "biliblanket," to break down the bilirubin in the skin. Usually, the baby is left to lay alone for this treatment. But the mother can hold the baby instead, and wear eye protectors herself. If they do not provide them, find sunglasses and wear those. Exposing the baby to sunlight through a window (unclothed) can lower the bilirubin level effectively.

BEING PREPARED

The care providers need to know the mother's wishes for labor and birth. Therefore, when the mother is in labor, she knows that they are aware of what she wants and does not want. There are many "birth plan" templates on the Internet to print out and complete. Birth wishes can then be compiled into one to three pages, and given to those who will be in attendance. Give a copy in pregnancy to the care provider and birth team and have a few on hand to provide upon arrival to birthplace (if not birthing at home). Below are two samples of birth wishes.

BIRTH WISHES OF (your name here)

We are looking forward to sharing our birth experience with you. We would appreciate you reviewing the below. We understand there may be situations in which our choices may not be possible, but ask that you respect ALL of our wishes for us to have the best experience possible. We want to be informed of any procedures in advance, to give informed consent. My husband and my doula will be in attendance. As long as the baby and I are healthy, I do not want to discuss induction before 42 weeks.

LABOR

- ☐ I expect that doctors and hospital staff will discuss all procedures with me before they are performed.
- ☐ I want to labor freely in the room, walking, changing positions, and using the bathroom as needed or desired.
- ☐ I prefer to wear my clothes rather than a hospital gown.
- ☐ I prefer to eat and drink throughout labor as desired.
- ☐ I will remain hydrated by drinking moderate amounts of fluids. Please do not administer an IV or heparin lock unless an emergency.
- ☐ I want a quiet, soothing environment during labor, with dim lights and minimal interruptions.
- ☐ I may want to play music.
- ☐ I wish for minimal to no vaginal exams. Please ask first, I will decide.
- ☐ I would rather have a tear than an episiotomy and neither if possible.
- ☐ I may vocalize as desired during labor and ask for no comments or criticism regarding this.
- ☐ I do not want continuous fetal monitoring. As long as the baby is doing well, I prefer that fetal heart tones be monitored intermittently with an external monitor or doppler, even if the membranes have ruptured.
- ☐ Please do not permit observers such as interns, students, or additional staff into the room without my permission.
- ☐ I want to avoid induction and artificial rupture of membranes.
- ☐ Please do not offer me drugs (Pitocin, epidural, narcotics, anesthesia).

☐ If I ask for pain relief, please feel free to offer nonmedical choices for coping or remind me how close I am to the birth.

PUSHING/BIRTHING STAGE

☐ Even if I am fully dilated, and assuming the baby is not in distress, I want to wait to feel an urge to push before beginning the pushing phase.

☐ I prefer to push or not push according to my instincts and would prefer not to have guidance or coaching in this effort.

☐ I do not want to use stirrups while pushing.

☐ I wish to birth in any position I like.

☐ I want a mirror available in case I want to see head crowning.

☐ I may want to touch my baby's head as it crowns.

☐ I want a soothing environment during the actual birth, with dim lights and quiet voices.

☐ If the gender of the baby is unknown, please do not call out the baby's gender.

☐ I want my husband to help catch the baby.

IMMEDIATELY AFTER BIRTH

☐ Place baby on my stomach/chest for direct skin to skin, and for the first several hours to help regulate baby's body temperature. I will hold baby through delivery of the placenta and any repairs.

☐ DO NOT CLAMP THE CORD, OR CUT IT UNTIL I SAY SO. I wish to wait until placenta is delivered or the baby and I are ready for it to happen.

☐ I want to breastfeed the baby immediately. Please do not give the baby supplements (including formula, glucose, plain water, or pacifier).

☐ I want a lactation consultant to visit my room at some point.

☐ I prefer to wait for spontaneous delivery of the placenta and do not want a routine injection of Pitocin.

☐ Please show me the placenta after it is delivered. I plan to keep it and would like it placed in a container to take home.

☐ Please evaluate baby at my bedside, on my abdomen. Do not take him/her away to weigh, footprints, etc. Please do not bathe my baby.

☐ If the baby must go to the nursery for evaluation or medical treatment, I or my husband will accompany the baby at all times.

☐ Please delay eye medication for the baby for several hours after the birth. I want it administered while baby is on my chest. If available, I would prefer erythromycin eye treatment or other antibiotic eye drops instead of silver nitrate. (if you want this) If not: I would like to waive the administration of eye antibiotics. OR I would prefer to have Vitamin K administered orally. OR I would like to waive the administration of routine Vitamin K unless medically indicated.

☐ I defer the PKU screening and all vaccinations, including Hepatitis B.

ᔇ

ONE SHEET BIRTH WISHES OF _____

Thank you for being a part of my birthing experience. I ask that these wishes be honored as best they can. I want to give informed consent.

☐ I will have my husband and doula in attendance.

☐ Lights turned low

☐ Minimal cervical exams

☐ I wish to avoid taking any drugs in labor

☐ I want to birth in any position that I like

☐ I will push when it feels right

☐ Please keep voices low

☐ Do not clamp or cut the cord until 10 minutes after the baby's birth, or when I say

☐ Do not wipe the baby off after the birth. I want to leave on the vernix, blood, etc.

☐ Please hand baby to me immediately after birth, skin to skin

☐ Please take baby's vitals as I hold him/her

☐ I do not wish for weighing and such to be done until 5 hours after the birth

☐ I want to deliver the placenta spontaneously, without drugs, with an hour to do so

LABOR ENTICING/INDUCING METHODS

To avoid medical induction, women have found the following things can encourage labor to begin, including but not limited to: sexual intercourse, nipple stimulation, essential oils, walking, dancing, eating pineapple, spicy foods, drinking castor oil, and acupuncture or acupressure from a skilled practitioner. The following are additional options that have been utilized to get labor going, the cervix opened, etc.

It is essential to study these techniques further if planning to use them. You will find both non-medical and medical induction methods listed below.

ACUPUNCTURE

Acupuncture has been used in China to reduce pain in labor, to augment or increase labor contractions, and for other birth-related reasons, for more than 2000 years. The earliest evidence of the use of acupuncture dates back to the Stone Age, around 3000 BC. In this traditional Chinese medicine, Qi is an energy that flows through the body along 14 different paths. Miniscule acupuncture needles are inserted into specific points along those pathways to stimulate energy and blood. At the end of pregnancy, acupuncture can help the cervix become more ripe and ready for labor, and can relax the mother, allowing the body to be in a state of openness.

ACCUPRESSURE

There are major acupressure points that may induce labor, augment labor, ease pain, etc. Make sure to consult someone knowledgeable before performing. The most common points are:

- **Bladder 32 point (BL32)** is used to get contractions started. B32 is in the dimple at the base of the back, above the buttocks. Use the thumb to press firmly. Massage for a few minutes, moving down towards the buttocks.

- **Spleen 6 point (SP6)** can also help labor move a little faster. Located on the back of the calf, about 2 inches above the inner lower ankle bone. Apply firm continuous pressure with the index finger for a few seconds, wait a minute, and then repeat.

- **Bladder 60 point (BL60)** is used to induce labor, ease pain, and help with malposition. It is in the space between the ankle bone and Achilles tendon. Use your thumb to lightly massage BL60 for a few minutes.

- **Pericardium 8 point (PC8)** is often called "labor palace" because of its effectiveness at starting contractions. It is in the middle of the palm. If you make a fist, it's where the tip of your middle finger touches your palm. Use the thumb of the other hand to apply light pressure and gently massage for a few seconds.

- **Bladder 67 point (BL67)** is can trigger contractions and encourage babies to turn. It is on the outer edge of the pinky toe, where the nail bed starts. Use the thumb and index finger to firmly pinch it.

- **Large intestine 4 point (LI4)** known as Hegu, meaning "joining valley," can also lessen first stage labor pains. It is located on the outside of the hand, deep between the webbing of the thumb and pointer finger, right below the pointer finger knuckle. Use the thumb of the other hand to massage using soft pressure. Massage for a minute, wait a minute, and repeat.

- **Gallbladder 21 point (GB21)** Some practitioners recommend against using it during pregnancy precisely because it can induce labor. It can also reduce pain when used during contractions. It is located in the middle of the shoulder muscle, above the collarbone. Use the pointer finger and thumb to firmly pinch it, then massage with downward pressure for a few seconds.

- **Kidney 1 (KID1)** point pulls energy downward and is typically useful in the transition phase of labor. It can be calming and help with stress or anxiety. It is located in the center sole of the foot in the depression next to the ball of the foot.

LABOR INDUCING MASSAGE
Certain massage techniques and trigger points can help induce labor. Massage also relaxes the mother, which can help with dilation and release the necessary hormones to begin labor.

NIPPLE STIMULATION
When the mother's nipples are manually stimulated, whether through touch or a breast pump, oxytocin is released, which facilitates uterine contractions. The mother or her partner can focus on one breast at a time for 15 minutes. A natural oil can be used to lubricate.

CASTOR OIL
Castor oil is a powerful laxative, also known as Oleum Palmae Christi, from the seeds of the Ricinus communis plant. Reports dating back to ancient Egypt note it as a labor-inducing technique. Usually, 2 ounces are taken in 24 hours, in the morning hours, and mixed with orange juice. The results of castor oil inducing labor are mixed; it can cause cramping and diarrhea, and when effective at kicking off labor, can cause irregular and painful contractions, which can stress mom and baby alike, and lead to exhaustion or dehydration. It may also cause the baby to pass meconium, or their first stool, before birth.

FOLEY BULB
A Foley bulb induction involves inserting a Foley catheter, a long rubber tube with an inflatable balloon on one end, into the cervix, and filling it with air or sterile water. When the balloon inflates inside the cervix, it puts pressure on the cervical cells, assists dilation, and increases the tissue's response to prostaglandins and oxytocin. It is a safe procedure, with no evidence of increased risks for infection.

CERVIDIL
Cervidil is a medication used in a hospital setting for women having a healthy pregnancy who are on or past their guess date. It is used to help soften, relax, and ripen the cervix, encouraging dilation. A Cervidil insert is like a tampon and contains dinoprostone, a prostaglandin that the body naturally

makes in preparation for labor. The mother is monitored for changes in her cervix, signs of active labor, and the baby's condition. It stays inside anywhere from 1–12 hours, and sometimes a second insert is applied.

Some common side effects associated with this drug are: diarrhea, fever, nausea, vomiting, stomach cramps. Also possible: low blood pressure, slow heart rate, chills, pain in the lower abdomen, foul-smelling vaginal discharge, increase in bleeding of the uterus, fetal heart rate abnormality, uterine hyperstimulation (with or without fetal distress), and fetal distress without uterine hyperstimulation. Consider these risks and the other options mentioned above.

CYTOTEC

Cytotec (misoprostol) is often used to induce labor and ripen the cervix despite being classified by the FDA as a Pregnancy Category X drug, due to studies that have demonstrated fetal abnormalities, and evidence of fetal risk. The adverse reactions associated with the use of Cytotec in labor, as found on its label, include: birth defects, premature birth, abortion, uterine hyperstimulation, uterine rupture, hysterectomy or surgery to remove fallopian tubes and ovaries, amniotic fluid embolism, severe vaginal bleeding (hemorrhaging), retained placenta, shock, fetal bradycardia, pelvic pain, and potential maternal mortality or fetal death.

The original manufacturer of Cytotec issued a letter in 2000 to healthcare professionals across the country stating: "Cytotec administration by any route is contraindicated in women who are pregnant because it can cause abortion. Cytotec is not approved for the induction of labor or abortion." The Tatia Oden French Memorial Foundation was formed by a grieving mother, whose daughter Tatia, a healthy 32 year old, when birthing her first child, was given Cytotec because she was a little under 42 weeks pregnant. Ten hours after it was administered, both she and her baby died. The foundation gives women complete information concerning medical interventions and drugs administered during childbirth. Their website is tatia.org. Do not take Cytotec to induce labor.

SWEEPING THE MEMBRANES

A doctor or midwife inserts a gloved finger through the cervical canal and uses a sweeping motion to gently lift the amniotic sac, or fetal membrane, from the cervix and lower part of the uterus. This technique releases prostaglandins, which are chemicals that help soften and open the cervix. The cervix must be dilated at least one centimeter for this procedure. Mothers agree it is rather painful, and possible effects are: irregular contractions, bleeding, waters breaking, formal induction, and longer labors.

BREAKING THE WATERS

This procedure is called an amniotomy or artificial rupture of membranes (AROM). The doctor or midwife will perform a careful vaginal exam to make sure the baby's head is firmly applied to the cervix. The membranes will be snagged using an amnihook (a large device with a small sharp end, similar to a crochet hook) or an amnicot (a glove with a small sharp hook at the end of one finger). After creating a tear in the bag, the amniotic fluid will begin to flow out. There are contraindications in which amniotomy should not be done, such as abnormal presentation or if the baby's head is not engaged. Discuss with care provider if it is a viable and intelligent option.

Also, know the risks of AROM, which include: failure of labor to start, increase in fetal malposition, cord prolapse, fetal distress, increased chance of C-section.

Before agreeing to have the waters broken, ask the doctor or midwife:
- Will I be allowed to walk after my water is broken?
- Will I need extra monitoring?
- What signs of problems will you be looking for, and how?
- How would you guess doing this will change labor in my case?
- Are there other interventions that may be needed because of this?
- What are my alternatives?
- Do I have time to make this decision?

ASSESSMENT

Often, if a mother is past the "due date," the care provider may ask to perform a cervical exam to assist in predicting if spontaneous labor is indeed imminent (known as a cervix score or Bishops Score). The following factors are taken into consideration:

CERVICAL POSITION (posterior, middle, anterior)

The position of the cervix changes with menstrual cycles and also tends to become more anterior (nearer the opening of the vagina) as labor approaches.

CERVICAL CONSISTENCY (firm, medium, soft)

In women pregnant for the first time, the cervix is typically tougher and resistant to stretching, much like a balloon that has not been previously inflated (it feels like the bottom of a chin). With subsequent vaginal deliveries, the cervix becomes softer.

CERVICAL EFFACEMENT (0–30%, 40–50%, 60–70%, 80–100%)

Effacement translates to how 'thin' the cervix is. The cervix is normally approximately three centimeters long. The cervix will efface until it is paper thin, or 'fully effaced'.

CERVICAL DILATION (Closed, 1–2 cm, 3–4 cm, 5–10)

Dilation is a measure of how open the hole is, and an indicator of progression in the first stage of labor.

FETAL STATION (–2, –3, –1/0, +1/+2)

Fetal station describes the position of the fetus's head in relation to the distance from the ischial spines, which are approximately 3–4 cm inside the vagina and not usually felt. Health professionals visualize where they are and use them as a reference point. Negative numbers indicate that the head is further inside than the ischial spines and positive numbers show that the head is below the level of the ischial spines.

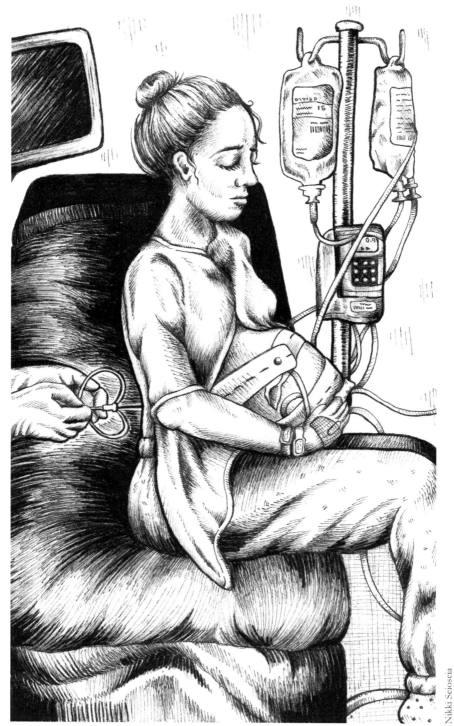

Nikki Scioscia

CHAPTER 11:
RISKS OF INTERVENTIONS

"The knowledge of how to give birth without outside interventions lies deep within each woman. Successful childbirth depends on the acceptance of the process."
- SUZANNE ARMS

"Birth is as safe as life gets."
- HARRIETTE HARTIGAN

"Many women have described their experiences of childbirth as being associated with a spiritual uplifting, the power of which they have never previously been aware. To such a woman, childbirth is a monument of joy within her memory. She turns to it in thought to seek again an ecstasy which passed too soon."
- GRANTLY DICK READ,
Childbirth Without Fear

To INTERVENE MEANS TO modify, to come between, or to interfere with the outcome or course of events. Intervening may be necessary; we do it if someone plans to harm him or herself, or if we want to prevent calamity from occurring. But when there is no need, intervening can cause more damage than good. Risks should be weighed heavily, especially in the case of labor and birth, as the chemistry and physiology that is present in both mother and baby are mysterious and purposeful. Trying to control something that is orchestrated so well by the human bodies, hormones, love, and unseen forces will inevitably bring less than optimal outcomes. "Primum non nocere" means "first of all, do no harm," is a principal precept students are taught in medical school and a fundamental principle in the world. Originally stated by Hippocrates, it is a way of saying, it may be better not to do something, than to risk causing more harm than good.

INTERVENTIONS

75% of American women will receive an epidural for the birth of their child. Which means that 75% of the babies coming into the world will also receive an epidural. A pregnant mother should have access to solid information to guide her choices, know the risks associated with these procedures and be encouraged to trust herself, her body, and her intuition. The following interventions will be addressed in this chapter:

Induction: stimulating uterine contractions to accomplish delivery prior to the onset of spontaneous labor

Pitocin: the artificial oxytocin hormone used to induce labor

Epidural: a local anesthetic—still derived from cocaine—that is injected into the space around the tough coverings that protect the spinal cord.

INDUCTION

Induction of labor refers to techniques for stimulating uterine contractions to accomplish delivery prior to the onset of spontaneous labor. It is one of the most commonly performed obstetrical procedures in the United States. Induction comes with increased risk for mother and baby, such as post partum hemorrhage, hyper-stimulation of the uterus (where the uterus contracts too frequently, decreasing blood flow to the baby), the use of extra interventions such as continuous fetal monitoring, the need for additional pain relief, and a failed induction leading to a Cesarean.

Electively induced labor more than doubles the risk of C-section compared to spontaneous labor. The risk of maternal death is five times higher in a C-section. The risk is more than tripled when cervical ripening medication is used. Around 15% of inductions require an assisted birth such as a forceps. Being induced can increase the length of labor. Induction and cesarean both lead to an increased risk of infection. "Surgical site infection (SSI) is one of the most common complications following cesarean section, and has an incidence of 3%–15%." (*International Journal of Women's Health*, Postcesarean wound infection: prevalence, impact, prevention, and management challenges, Sivan Zuarez-Easton, Noah Zafran, [...], and Raed Salim, 2017)

Between 1990 and 2012, the overall frequency of labor induction more than doubled in the United States, rising from 9.5 to 23.3 percent, and early term (in the 37th and 38th week of gestation) inductions quadrupled, rising from 2 to 8 percent over a similar period of time. In 2009, The American College of Obstetrics and Gynecology issued new guidelines on the when and how for induction, listing 39 weeks as the accepted time for elective induction, but urging care providers to first consider three significant factors: the values and preferences of the pregnant woman, the staffing and facility resources available (to assist longer labors), and the protocol for "failed" induction.

"DUE DATES"

The estimated due date (EDD) can be off by up to two weeks, since most doctors, midwives, and online calculators use Naegele's rule to figure it out, which assumes a 28 day cycle, ovulating on day 14. To calculate the due date according to Naegele's rule, you add 7 days to the first day of your last period, and then count forward 9 months. This is akin to counting forward 280 days from your last period.

In 1744, Hermann Boerhaave, a professor from the Netherlands, came up with a formula for calculating due dates, with the basis being the records of 100 pregnant women. Boerhaave figured the EDD by adding 7 days to the last menstrual cycle, and then adding nine months. However, he did not explain whether you should add 7 days to the *first* day of the last period, or to the *last day* of the last period.

68 years later, Carl Naegele, a professor from Germany, quoted Boerhaave, and added his own thoughts. He, too, failed to say when to start counting, and his text can be interpreted one of two ways: either you add 7 days to the *first* day of the last cycle, or you add 7 days to the *last* day of the last cycle. As the 1800s went on, different doctors interpreted Naegele's rule in assorted ways, with most adding 7 days to the *last* day. But by the 1900s, American textbooks applied the view that added 7 days to the *first* day, and today, almost all doctors use this—a rule that is not based on any current evidence, and may not have even been intended by Naegele.

What shall be taken into consideration, is the following:

1. All women have different durations of their moon cycle; some have three days of bleeding and others five.
2. The time length of cycles is different; some have a 28-day-cycle and others 24 or 26.
3. The time of ovulation is different; some may ovulate on day 12, others day 14, etc.
4. The embryo may take longer to implant in the uterus for some.
5. Some babies may want to stay in the womb a little longer.

**A baby's brain at 35 weeks weighs
only two-thirds of what it will weigh
at 39 to 40 weeks**

     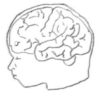

35 weeks   **39 to 40 weeks**

"GUESS MONTH"

A study was conducted in 2013, of 125 healthy mothers, where researchers knew the exact days each woman ovulated, conceived, and when implantation occurred. After excluding preterm births and pregnancy-related medical conditions, the median time from the first day of the last menstrual period to birth, for the remaining 113 women, was 40 weeks and 5 days after the last menstrual period.

What are thought to be 38 weeks could actually be 36. Or 40 weeks could actually be 38-1/2. Trust the baby to decide when he or she is ready to join the world. They are teaching patience and surrender. My midwife recommended that I tell friends and family a "guess month" rather than a "due" date. It was excellent advice. I would say, "Late October, early November," if anyone asked. My guess date was October 22. It was a relief to have no one hounding me or worrying about when the baby was *supposed* to come. He arrived October 27, at 40 weeks and 5 days.

∽

Please visit www.evidencebasedbirth.com to read wonderfully written articles about due dates by Rebecca Dekker, PhD, RN, APRN. Since this book will be printed, you will find more current (and extensive) research and data on her site.

PITOCIN

The mother and baby make chemical messages that assist with labor, birth, and breastfeeding. The primary three hormones of birth are: oxytocin, prolactin, and beta-endorphins. High levels of these hormones help the mother feel calm, nurturing, alert, attentive, euphoric, while stimulating contractions, moving baby down, opening the cervix, and promoting lactation and breastfeeding.

The synthetic form of the oxytocin hormone is called Pitocin (aka "pit"). It produces strong, painful contractions but doesn't produce any of the feel-good, bonding or pain-killing hormones of natural labor. Artificial oxytocin doesn't cross the blood-brain barrier, and does not act in the same way as natural oxytocin does. Experts believe induced labor is more painful than a labor that starts naturally.

The two primary reasons obstetricians use Pitocin:

1. To induce birth in pregnant women who are "post-term", *i.e.* past 42 weeks gestation (known as "induction")
2. To speed up labor (known as "augmentation")

INDUCTION

Induction with pitocin can be a lifesaving intervention, and necessary in some circumstances to protect the well being of both the newborn and mother, but the use of routine induction today is excessive.

In 2013, the American College of Obstetricians and Gynecologists defined "full term" as week 39 through the end of week 41 of gestation; "early term" as week 37 through the end of week 38, and "late term" as week 42 and beyond. Mothers who go past the "due date" and even before they reach the date, may likely be encouraged to "get induced." I've heard mothers with a scheduled induction comment that their partner could then choose his time off, the grandparents were coming into town so they needed to have the baby by that date, or that they are just "over being pregnant." These are not medical reasons for stimulating the uterus, and although they may seem convenient for the outsiders, the insider (baby) may not be ready and willing. Inducing labor way before the baby and mother's body are ready can lead to uterine overstimulation, failure of induction, increased chance of cesarean birth, and fetal distress.

Accurate pregnancy dating is crucial to the diagnosis and management of post term pregnancy. Routine induction at 39 weeks, 40 weeks and 41 weeks is a practice that is often based in fear, and primarily pushed as a preventative of stillbirth. Vicki Flenady, director of the Center of Research Excellence in Stillbirth at the University of Queensland in Australia states, "There are some circumstances where women need to be induced or have a cesarean section before their due date. It's ideal if women reach their full gestation of 41 weeks, as this allows the baby to fully develop, especially in brain growth, which is very rapid towards the end of pregnancy."

"The perinatal mortality rate, defined as stillbirths plus early neonatal deaths, at 42 weeks of gestation is twice as high as that at term (4–7 versus 2–3 per 1000 deliveries, respectively). It increases 4-fold at 43 weeks and 5–7-fold at 44 weeks." (Bakketeig and Bergsjo, Effective Care in Pregnancy and Childbirth, 1989, Post-term pregnancy) Therefore, once at or past 42 weeks, induction would be a stronger consideration for the mother, and monitoring movement and receiving ultrasound is useful technology that can be employed. "It is believed that utero-placental insufficiency, meconium aspiration, and intrauterine infection are the underlying causes of the increased perinatal mortality rates in these cases." (Hannah ME, Fetal Maternal Medical Review 1993;5:3). Other potential causes include maternal diabetes, maternal obesity, pneumonia in the newborn, trauma, umbilical cord issues, and high blood pressure.

As many as 80% of women who reach 42 weeks gestation have an "unfavorable cervix," which means that an exam reveals the cervix has not yet dilated, softened, and thinned out much. The position of the baby in the canal is also a factor (fetal station). I worked with a mother who, at 42 weeks, was given the "unfavorable" news. She was admitted to the hospital early morning, requested and received the Foley bulb technique, and later an insertion of Cervadil (see previous chapter for non-medical and medical induction options). Twelve hours later, the insertion came out, and she went into active labor, birthing her child about 2 hours later, in a fast and intense birth.

AUGMENTATION

The problem with speeding up labor with pitocin is that it produces an abnormal labor. Synthetic oxytocin interferes with the delicate orchestration of the mother's natural occurring hormones during birth, and according to research, with the baby's hormones and brain as well. Contractions with Pitocin are stronger and closer together than normal contractions, due to a steady stream via IV, whereas the natural oxytocin produced by the brain comes in waves. Because Pitocin-induced contractions last longer, there is no time for the mother to recover in between. Chris Kresser, M.S. who has written many excellent articles on Natural Childbirth says:

> "This can cause significant stress to the baby because there's not enough time to recover from the reduced blood flow that happens when the placenta is compressed with each contraction. It can deprive the baby of necessary supplies of blood and oxygen, which can in turn lead to abnormal fetal heart rate patterns and fetal distress."

You can find the full article, "Natural Childbirth VI: Pitocin Side Effects and Risks" and more, at www.chriskresser.com

〰

So many times I have heard mothers say they had to have a C-section because the "baby's heart rate dropped." Birth activist Doris Haire describes the effects of synthetic oxytocin on the baby as follows: "The situation is analogous to holding an infant under the surface of the water, allowing the infant to come to the surface to gasp for air, but not to breathe."

The U.S. Pitocin package insert warns that the drug can cause:

- Fetal heart abnormalities (slow heart beat, PVCs and arrhythmias)
- Low APGAR scores
- Neonatal jaundice
- Neonatal retinal hemorrhage
- Permanent central nervous system or brain damage
- Fetal death

A study in Sweden showed a roughly 3 times greater risk of asphyxia (oxygen deprivation) for babies born after augmentation with Pitocin. A study in Nepal showed that induced babies were 5 times more likely to have signs of brain damage at birth. There has been speculation that Pitocin may have an association to the development of autism.

Evidence shows that women who receive this drug have increased risk of postpartum hemorrhage, likely due to the prolonged exposure to non-pulsed oxytocin. This makes the oxytocin receptors in her uterus insensitive to oxytocin ("oxytocin resistance") and her own post birth oxytocin release ineffective in preventing hemorrhage. According to one study, participants who were induced with Pitocin had a 300-fold decrease of the oxytocin receptor gene in the uterine muscle when compared to receptor availability in non-induced labor.

Pitocin affects the natural hormonal cascade, which is important for a smooth, gentle, undisturbed birth. In one study, women who received Pitocin to speed up labor did not experience an increase in beta-endorphin levels.

Hormonal disruption explains the reduced rate of breastfeeding following labor induced with Pitocin. Also, bonding and breastfeeding go hand in hand. If the bonding (chemically, physically and emotionally) is not strong during birth, the bonding needed for breastfeeding may wane as well. The baby's experience of being rushed and not having their timing honored, may also contribute. As Sunni Karll writes, "If someone yanks us out of a place intrusively, we naturally recoil and go within in order to maintain balance against this outside force. The difference of being "received" compared to being "forced" results in opening to this world or shielding ourselves from it."

EPIDURAL

The first physician to use an epidural was a neurologist in New York named Dr. Leonard J. Corning. In 1885 he injected cocaine into the back of a patient suffering from spinal weakness and seminal incontinence.

Today, epidurals are the most popular method of labor pain relief in U.S. hospitals. 75 percent of American mothers get an epidural.

In an epidural, a local anesthetic—still derived from cocaine—is injected into the space around the tough coverings that protect the spinal cord. A thin tube is inserted so a dose can be given over a period of time. Epidurals block nerve signals from both the motor and sensory nerves, which provides pain relief but immobilizes the lower part of the recipient's body. Traditional epidurals take about 10–20 minutes to work.

Epidurals, like Pitocin, largely interfere with the body's superb natural hormone orchestration, and inhibit beta-endorphin production, which then prohibits the altered state of awareness or consciousness-shift experienced in undisturbed birth. Epidurals reduce the production and increase of oxytocin during labor, and blunt the oxytocin peak/high that occurs at the time of birth because the stretching receptors of a woman's lower vagina are numbed. As Dr. Sarah Buckley explains: "A woman laboring with an epidural therefore misses out on the final powerful contractions of labor and must use her own effort, often against gravity, to compensate for this loss. This explains the increased length of the second stage of labor and the increased need for forceps when an epidural is used."

Epidurals have been shown to hinder catecholamine production. Catecholamine can slow or stop labor in the early stages. But in the second stage of labor, it promotes the fetus ejection reflex. Therefore, inhibiting catecholamine production may make delivery more taxing and contribute to the baby having a difficult time navigating the way out, or getting "stuck."

Epidurals limit the release of prostaglandin F2 alpha, a lipid compound that stimulates uterine contractions and is thought to be involved with the initiation of labor. During an undisturbed labor, prostaglandin F2 alpha levels should naturally increase. One study revealed that women with epidurals experienced a decrease in PGF2 alpha and an increase in labor length from 4.7 to 7.8 hours.

WHAT ARE SOME POSSIBLE CONTENTS OF AN EPIDURAL?

Epidural medications fall into a class of drugs called local anesthetics, such as bupivacaine, chloroprocaine, or lidocaine. They are often delivered in combination with opioids or narcotics such as fentanyl and sufentanil, to decrease the required dose of local anesthetic. These may be used in combination with epinephrine, fentanyl, morphine, or clonidine to prolong the epidural's effect or to stabilize the mother's blood pressure.

*Note: Please feel free to research these drugs more. Here are some things I read and felt compelled to share.

Depending on the route of administration, local anesthetics are distributed to some extent to all body tissues, with high concentrations found in organs such as the liver, lungs, heart, and brain.

BUPIVACAINE

Bupivacaine crosses the placenta and is a pregnancy category C drug. However, it is approved for use at term in obstetrical anesthesia. Bupivacaine is excreted in breast milk. Risks of discontinuing breastfeeding versus discontinuing bupivacaine should be discussed with the patient.

CHLOROPROCAINE

Following systemic absorption, toxic blood concentrations of local anesthetics can produce central nervous system stimulation, depression, or both. Apparent central stimulation may be manifested as restlessness, tremors and shivering, which may progress to convulsions. Local anesthetics have a primary depressant effect on the medulla and on higher centers. The depressed stage may occur without a prior stage of central nervous system stimulation.

ROPIVACAINE /NAROPIN

A local anaesthetic, that when injected, makes the nerves nearby unable to pass messages to the brain and therefore prevents or relieves pain. Often used in C-sections operations. "Breathing, blood pressure, oxygen levels, and other vital signs will be watched closely while you are receiving ropivacaine. Call the doctor if you have joint pain or stiffness, or weakness in any part of your body that occurs after your surgery, even months later." Warning on package: Tell your doctor if you are pregnant, are breastfeeding, or intend to breast-feed. Naropin is not recommended for children under 12 years of age.

LIDOCAINE

Common side effects with intravenous use include sleepiness, muscle twitching, confusion, changes in vision, numbness, tingling, and vomiting. It can cause low blood pressure and an irregular heart rate.

FENTANYL

Belongs to a group of medicines called narcotic analgesics. It is a powerful drug used to relieve pain. It works by changing the way your brain receives pain messages. Naropin with Fentanyl is a combination of the two drugs and produces anaesthesia (loss of feeling) and analgesia (pain relief).

SUFENTANIL

Sufentanil is a synthetic opioid analgesic that is five to 10 times more potent than its analogue, fentanyl and 1000 times more potent than morphine. It is currently marketed for intravenous and epidural anesthesia and analgesia.

✍

I have heard a male anesthesiologist say to a mother before administering an epidural, "This is not going to change anything. It's just going to make everything better." It most definitely changes things. I have heard "This won't pass onto your baby." A statement that is also false. Any drug that a woman uses during labor enters the body of the child. The cells, tissues, bloodstream, atoms, molecules, energy, psychology, spirit, and breath must all be taken into consideration. The body is not separated into parts. It is a whole. Lying to the mother, as well as not letting her know the risks, is irresponsible and disrespectful.

As Kesser states, "As is the case with all medical interventions, it's important to critically examine the balance between benefit and risk—especially when we're talking about the use of powerful drugs with otherwise healthy pregnant mothers and their babies."

EPIDURALS HAVE BEEN SHOWN TO HAVE THE FOLLOWING EFFECTS:

- They lengthen labor.
- They triple the risk of severe perineal tear.
- They may increase the risk of cesarean section by 2.5 times.
- They triple the occurrence of induction with synthetic oxytocin (Pitocin).
- They quadruple the chances a baby will be persistently posterior (POP, face up) in the final stages of labor, which in turn decreases the chances of spontaneous vaginal birth.
- They decrease the chances of spontaneous vaginal delivery. In 6 of 9 studies reviewed in one analysis, less than half of women who received an epidural had a spontaneous vaginal delivery.
- Epidural makes pushing more difficult and additional medications or interventions may be needed, such as forceps, increasing the chances of complications from instrumental delivery. When women with an epidural had a forceps delivery, the amount of force used by the clinician was almost double that used when an epidural was not in place. This is significant because instrumental deliveries can increase the short-term risks of bruising, facial injuries, displacement of skull bones and blood clots in the scalp for babies, and of episiotomy and tears to the vagina and perineum in mothers.
- They increase the risk of pelvic floor problems (urinary, anal and sexual disorders) in mothers after birth, which rarely resolve spontaneously.
- Epidurals may cause the mother's blood pressure to suddenly drop. Therefore, blood pressure will be routinely checked to help ensure adequate blood flow to your baby. If there is a sudden drop in blood pressure, mother may need to be treated with IV fluids, medications, and oxygen.
- Possible severe headache caused by leakage of spinal fluid. Less than 1% of women experience this, but if symptoms persist, a procedure called a "blood patch", an injection of your blood into the epidural space, can be performed to relieve the headache.
- After an epidural is placed, the mother will need to alternate sides while lying in bed and have continuous monitoring for changes in fetal heart rate. Lying in one position can sometimes cause labor to slow down or stop.

- Possible side effects: shivering, a ringing of the ears, backache, soreness where the needle is inserted, nausea, vomiting, or difficulty urinating.
- For a few hours after the birth, the lower half of the mother's body may feel numb.
- In rare instances, permanent nerve damage may result in the area where the catheter was inserted.

EPIDURAL EFFECTS ON BABIES:

- Drugs administered by epidural enter the baby's bloodstream at equal and sometimes even higher levels than those present in the mother's bloodstream.
- Because babies' immune systems are immature, it takes longer for them to eliminate epidural drugs. For example, the half-life of bupivacaine, a commonly used epidural analgesic, is 2.7 hours in an adult but close to 8 hours in a newborn. Studies have found detectable amounts of bupivacain metabolites in the urine of exposed newborns for 36 hours following spinal anesthesia for cesareans.
- Some studies have found deficits in newborn abilities that are consistent with the known toxicity of drugs used in epidurals. Other studies have found that local anesthetics used in epidurals may adversely affect the newborn immune system, possibly by activating the stress response.
- There is evidence that epidurals can compromise fetal blood and oxygen supply, probably via the decrease in maternal blood pressure that epidurals are known to cause.
- Studies suggest that some babies will have trouble "latching on" causing breastfeeding difficulties.
- Baby might experience: respiratory depression, fetal malpositioning, and an increase in fetal heart rate variability, thus increasing the need for forceps, vacuum, cesarean deliveries, and episiotomy.

〜

Following is information that women are currently given (unless they aren't) if considering an epidural for pain relief. This is best received and read by mothers prior to labor, instead of during labor.

EPIDURAL ANESTHESIA EXPECTED RESULTS

A temporary decrease or loss of feeling and or movement to lower part of the body, which may provide relief from pain during a prolonged or difficult labor. This type of anesthesia/analgesia does not alter the mental status as occurs with IV or injection pain medications. Occasionally the anesthesia does not completely take away the pain, or only provides numbness on one side.

Technique—Medication is injected through a needle, and a catheter is placed outside the spinal canal in the epidural space.

RISKS FOR MOTHER:
- High spinal block: You could experience shortness of breath, respiratory depression or respiratory/cardiac arrest. You may need an emergency cesarean section and resuscitation.
- Adverse reaction to anesthetic agent: May lead to respiratory paralysis, cardiac arrest, brain damage, heart attack, convulsions, stroke or death.

RISKS FOR BABY:
- Reduced blood supply to the placenta may cause fetal distress, brain damage, or death.

OTHER CONSIDERATIONS:
- Continuous electronic fetal monitoring will be used to check for signs of fetal stress. Epidural anesthesia/analgesia may cause slow, less effective labor contractions. Pitocin may have to be added to the IV to stimulate stronger contractions.
- More epidural medicine may be needed to relieve the pain of stronger Pitocin induced contractions. Pitocin can cause more risk to the baby. Arrested labor may result in cesarean section, which is a major abdominal surgery and poses increased risk for the mother.
- If an epidural is given in early labor, it increases the chance that the baby is in the wrong position as it comes into the pelvis. This may increase the need for a cesarean delivery.

- Epidural anesthesia decreases the mother's ability to push and increases the need for forceps, vacuum, or cesarean section. Forceps or vacuum assisted deliveries have a greater need for an episiotomy and deep tears into the perineal muscle. This can increase the pain and healing time after giving birth.
- Back strain or injury to the hips and knees may occur due to the inability to feel if the body is in an awkward position.
- The mother cannot respond naturally to labor cues, and may not feel as much control over the birth process.
- You will not be able to walk around, or use the tub, shower, or toilet.
- The epidural may cause the mother's temperature to rise, requiring additional tests for you and the baby to evaluate for possible infections.
- You may need a catheter inserted into your bladder if you are unable to urinate.
- You will be limited to a clear liquid diet only after an epidural because of increased surgical risk if a cesarean is needed.
- You will be monitored often for vital signs after an epidural, so a blood pressure cuff will be placed on your arm, a pulse oximeter will be placed on a finger, and you will receive intravenous fluids.

POSTPARTUM EFFECTS:

- Epidurals may cause severe headaches, migraines, temporary or permanent nerve damage, muscle weakness in legs, numbness or tingling sensation, and long-term backache.

NEWBORN EFFECTS:

The epidural may decrease the newborn baby's ability to nurse well for the first 12–72 hours.

_____All forms of anesthesia or medications have some risk, and rare unexpected complications other than what is listed here may occur.

_____I understand that it is my choice to choose the type of pain relief method I feel is appropriate for my baby's birth including an epidural, IV pain medications, or comfort measures as listed on my birth plan.

_____If I choose an epidural, I understand that every effort will be made to get an epidural administered in a timely manner. I understand an epidural may not be appropriate if the labor is advancing quickly and the procedure cannot be done safely.

_____If a cesarean delivery becomes necessary, the epidural may be adequate anesthesia for surgery but general anesthesia may be necessary if complete pain relief is not achieved.

_____I have had the opportunity to ask my OB physician or midwife questions regarding pain relief methods for labor and delivery.

_____I understand this is NOT A CONSENT FORM FOR THE PROCEDURE OF THE EPIDURAL, but is confirmation that I have been educated on the effects of an epidural which may affect the obstetrical care I receive from my physician or midwife. If I choose to have an epidural during my labor, the anesthesia provider who will be administering the epidural will also inform me of risks associated with the procedure.

Please initial the above statements, and sign below.
Patient Signature _____ **Date**_____
OB Provider Signature_____ **Date**_____

CONTINUOUS FETAL MONITORING

Many mothers who are birthing in hospitals are told that it is routine, policy, or protocol, to be hooked up to an electronic fetal monitor continuously while in labor and birthing. I had a mother tell me her doctor said it was hospital policy. The mother was not high risk. So I called the hospital, and had them read the requirements to be considered high risk, thereby warranting the continuous monitoring. The mother went back to the doctor and relayed the information given by the hospital. I cannot recall the doctor's response, but I do recall that the mother did not have continuous monitoring during her birth.

Because monitors have long been two belts (one for mother and one for baby) that move around and can be bothersome to the mother; these days, bluetooth monitors are becoming popular, with medical staff touting that it gives mothers more freedom to move. My concern is, what effect does it have on the baby? Bluetooth devices emit Radio Frequency (RF) Radiation, which is the same radiation a microwave uses to cook food. There are hundreds of scientific studies that link RF Radiation to cancer. The World Health Organization has classified it as a possible "carcinogen."

Constant fetal monitoring is used so that hospitals have a record of the entire labor. I believe it has to do with the fear of lawsuits, so that there can be evidence of "non-reassuring fetal heart tones," which is the "second most common reason for first-time Cesareans (23%) after Failure to Progress (34%)," according to a joint consensus of the American College of Obstetricians and Gynecologists and the Society for Maternal-Fetal Medicine. Induction, augmentation, and epidural can contribute tremendously to non-reassuring heart tones, as noted in this chapter.

PITOCIN AFTER BIRTH

I have seen mothers birth their baby unmedicated, and are then told it is "standard," "policy," or "required," to receive an injection of Pitocin to prevent hemorrhage, even if her bleeding is a typical amount. If the mother agrees to receive the injection, oftentimes her legs will start shaking, and she will come down from the hormonal high, the natural chemistry in the body altered. The drug will travel into the breastmilk, and the baby may not respond well, possibly creating a hindrance in breastfeeding. If the bleeding is in fact abnormal, then the injection can be life-saving and crucial to prevent excessive blood loss.

A BENEFICIAL INTERVENTION

"In mothers with a history of herpes simplex virus, the administration of acyclovir for viral suppression is an important strategy to prevent genital herpetic outbreaks requiring cesarean delivery and asymptomatic viral shedding. Given the favorable benefit-risk profile for the administration of maternal acyclovir, efforts should be made to ensure that women with a history of genital herpes, even in the absence of an outbreak in the current pregnancy, are offered oral suppressive therapy within 3–4 weeks of anticipated delivery and at the latest, at or beyond 36 weeks of gestation. Cesarean delivery is not recommended for women with a history of herpes simplex virus infection but no active genital disease during labor." (Safe Prevention of the Primary Cesarean Delivery, ACOG & Society for Maternal-Fetal Medicine, March 2014)

A DRUG-FREE BEGINNING

Interventions are in some cases necessary, they exist and can be useful, of course. For instance, if the mother has extreme exhaustion and cannot continue laboring, an epidural could allow for rest, and strength upon waking. But, these drugs are being used so routinely, without enough consideration for both the baby and/or the mother's well being. A woman's lack of self-confidence in her ability to birth comes from negative impressions from films, television, friends, and generally from society's imposition of anxiety about birth. Fear of the unknown, impatience, and wanting total control lends to the staggering use of drugs in birth. These interventions do not ensure comfort. And why expect birth (life and death) to be comfortable?

Some discomfort is part of the passage into motherhood and the physiological change a woman is given in birthing her child. This cocktail of hormones happening in labor and birth are designed for the two of them, and are natural drugs. Oxytocin, the love hormone, is strong, so if women are feeling loved and cared for, they won't feel a desire for drugs. This current dynamic of pressuring laboring mothers to take drugs to numb them of feeling can decrease through deeper listening, greater understanding, patience, and compassion.

As Sunni Karll writes in *Making a Difference, A Blueprint for Harmony:*

> "The less hindered a birth is, the more opportunity there is to bond. The whole purpose of having an unmedicated, natural birth is to allow and support this experience of bonding. Bonding cannot happen when either baby or mom are medicated or in pain."

We can begin a new culture of birth, where babies are not forced out too early and drugged on their way into the world; mothers are not drugged while bringing their babies forth from their womb. With less fear and more encouragement and support, mothers will feel empowered to birth their babies with intuition and love, and to actually feel the entirety of hormones, incredible sensations, and the passage of their child into this realm. This will assist with bonding, less post partum depression, less traumatic births, and more connection to the source of where we all come from.

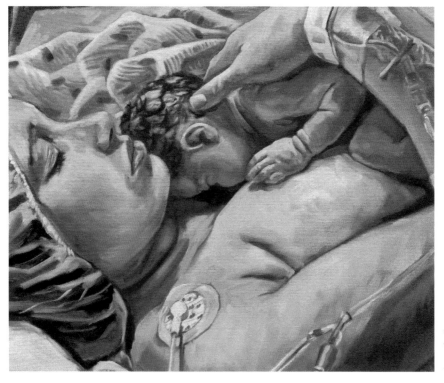

Amanda Greavette

CHAPTER 12:
CESAREAN OPERATION

*"A baby...you carry inside you for nine months, in your arms
for three years, and in your heart until the day you die."*
                                        - M A R Y   M A S O N

*"A healthy woman who delivers spontaneously
performs a job that cannot be improved upon."*
                              - A I D A N   M A C F A R L A N E
                              The Psychology of Childbirth

*"A pregnant woman is like a beautiful flowering tree, but take care
when it comes time for the harvest that you do not shake or bruise
the tree, for in doing so, you may harm both the tree and its fruit."*
                              - P E T E R   J A C K S O N ,   R N

CESAREAN SHOULD INDEED BE utilized in an emergency. But that is not entirely
what is going on in our time. I am in constant contact with pregnant women,
and I hear way too often that a C-section is being encouraged, scheduled,
or recommended to them, "Just to be safe." The rates are still rising, but
awareness is happening too. ACOG issued guidelines in 2016 stating that
pregnant women have the right to refuse treatment, including a C-section,
especially if it is not an emergency.

CESAREAN OPERATION
A cesarean is an operation by which a fetus is taken from the uterus by cutting
through the walls of the abdomen and uterus. Indeed they are sometimes
medically necessary; and when they are, can save the lives of mothers and
babies, which is something to be celebrated. However, a C-section is a serious,
major abdominal surgery, and the overuse of C-sections in the world present risks that outweigh the benefits. Since 1985, the international healthcare
community and the World Health Organization (WHO) have considered the

ideal rate for C-sections to be between 10–15% of all births. According to the Human Reproduction Program at the WHO, when a country's C-section rate is 10% or less, the number of maternal and newborn deaths decreases. When the rate goes above 10%, there is no evidence that mortality rates improve. In 1970, the C-section rate in the United States was roughly 5%; however 2015 data from the Center for Disease Control puts the U.S. rate at 32.7%. There is not enough medical evidence to prove that the number of C-sections performed in the United States is producing more benefit than risk.

A BRIEF HISTORY OF CESAREAN SECTION

(the following excerpt is from *Echoes from the Operating Room: Vignettes in Surgical History* by Carl R. Boyd, M.D.)

"Cesarean section is mentioned in the works of ancient folk-lore. The Greek god Apollo removed his son Asclepius from his mother's abdomen. The Roman book of Laws, named Lex Caesarea, required that the child be cut from the womb of a mother who died in childbirth. Religious edicts of the time required that the mother not be buried pregnant, and the mother and baby were buried in separate graves. This practice then became a measure of last resort to save the baby and not necessarily the mother's life, as the ability to save both the mother and the child would not become a routine possibility until the mid-nineteenth century.

The notion that the name Cesarean refers to the manner of birth of the Roman emperor Julius Caesar is false. Cesarean sections were performed in Roman times to save the baby, but there are no writings that document a mother surviving such a delivery, and Caesar's mother was alive to serve him as an advisor when he was emperor. The first written record of a mother and baby surviving a Cesarean section was from Switzerland in 1500 when Jacob Nufer, a pig castrator, performed the operation on his wife. Mrs. Nufer would go on to give birth vaginally to five more children, including twins. However, some seriously doubt the accuracy of this story.

The first successful Cesarean section in the United States of America occurred in Mason County, Virginia, in 1794. Dr. Jesse Bennett performed the procedure on his wife, Elizabeth. After the development of anesthesia, antisepsis, and asepsis, obstetricians began to improve the techniques employed in Cesarean section."

PRIMARY CESAREAN

A "primary cesarean" is a woman's first cesarean surgery. It is given that name because in the United States, once a woman has one, she is much more likely to birth all subsequent children via C-section. There are some disturbing trends about who ends up with a cesarean. A 2009 study on disparities in primary cesarean revealed that African American women were 25% more likely than white women to have a birth end in cesarean, while Hispanic women were 14% less likely than white women to birth by cesarean. The rates were adjusted for confounding factors, and there seemed to be no clear distinguishing variable other than race that accounted for the difference. African American women are also three to four times more likely to die from complications of childbirth than Caucasian women. According to a 2015 article in Scientific American, there is no explanation in the current medical research to explain African American women's increased risk of death related to childbirth, especially since the complications (most commonly preeclampsia and hemorrhage) that lead to death are the same complications, and occur at roughly the same rate, as those present in Caucasian women.

CESAREAN RATES THROUGHOUT THE WORLD

Recent statistics from 150 countries show a global C-section rate of 18.6% of all births—almost 1 in 5 women around the world will give birth via C-section.

HIGHEST C-SECTION RATES BY COUNTRY

(by Sam McCulloch Dip CBEd in Birth. Updated: June 5, 2018)

1. Dominican Republic: 56.4%
2. Brazil: 55.6% (public hospitals) 90% (private hospitals)
3. Eygpt, Turkey: 51%
4. China, Iran: 47%
5. Mexico, Chile: 45%

6. Republic of Korea, Romania, Italy: 36%
7. Hungary, Portugal, Poland: 35%
8. USA, Australia, Switzerland, Bulgaria: 33%
9. Germany, Sri Lanka, Albania, Slovac Republic: 30%
10. El Salvador, Argentina, Armenia: 29%
11. Austria, Luxemburg, Ireland: 28%
12. Canada, United Kingdom, Czech Republic: 26%
13. India: 18%
14. Finland, Iceland, Norway: 15%

In a study from March 2015, the highest rate of planned cesarean sections (before labor even began), aside from Brazil, was Greece at 38.8% and Italy at 25%. The lowest rates were in Finland (6.6%), the Netherlands (7.7%), and Norway (6.6%). In the U.K., planned cesarean rates were at 9%, Wales and Scotland 11%, and Northern Ireland 14.6%. Emergency C-section rates were highest in Romania at 33% and lowest in Sweden at 8.6%, where midwives oversee nearly all pregnancies.

THE TEN STATES IN THE USA WITH THE MOST CESAREANS
(according to the Center for Disease Control 2017 year)
1. Mississippi 37.8%
2. Louisiana 37.5%
3. Florida 37.2%
4. New Jersey 35.9%
5. West Virginia 35.2%
6. Kentucky 35.2%
7. Alabama 35.1%
8. Texas 35%
9. Connecticut 34.8%
10. Georgia 34.2%

WHY ARE THE CESAREAN RATES SO HIGH?

One reason for the high C-section rate, stated in an article in The Atlantic, is that "C-sections can be easily scheduled and quickly executed, so doctors schedule and bill as many as eight procedures a day rather than wait around for one or two natural births to wrap up." "It's likely three factors working together: financial, legal and technical," says Holly Kennedy, a professor of midwifery at the Yale School of Nursing. "As an obstetrician told me ... 'You're going to pay me more [to do a C-section], you're not going to sue me, and I'll be done in an hour, '" Kennedy says.

A mother once told me that after her child was pulled out of her uterus, the doctor said that in all her 40 years as an OBGYN, she had "never seen a baby fight so much to stay in" and that "the baby probably could have stayed another month." The C-section was done 9 days before her due date.

SEVERAL MORE REASONS FOR THE AMOUNT OF C-SECTIONS BEING DONE:

- Frequent use of epidural (75% in the USA)
- Unnecessary inductions & augmentation
- Medical malpractice concerns
- Convenience of the obstetrician or mother
- Due date fixation
- Lack of consistent prenatal care
- Increased maternal obesity
- Impatience/lack of support of doctors and nurses
- The increase in elective C-section deliveries
- Older women having babies told they are high-risk pregnancies
- Hospital infections
- Money
- Fear of birth and labor pain
- Cultural considerations such as birth date being lucky for future or destiny
- Belief that it is less traumatic to the baby and healthier for mom
- Belief that it prevents trauma and damage to the pelvic floor

THE TOP FACTORS THAT LEAD TO A CESAREAN

The most common indications for primary cesarean delivery include, in order of frequency: "failure to progress" in labor, abnormal fetal heart rate, an unfavorable position of the baby (such as breech or transverse), a pregnancy with multiples (twins/triplets, etc.), and a suspected "big baby," that is, a baby thought to weigh more than 11 pounds.

Some of these factors are easier to control than others. When it comes to failure to progress, there are many things a woman can do to help ensure that her labor progresses and does not stall. First, it is most beneficial for labor to begin spontaneously, or on its own. Induction of labor increases a woman's risk of cesarean section, so it is crucial to avoid any induction that is not medically required. Reaching your estimated due date is not a medical indication for induction! The average gestation for first-time mothers is 40 weeks plus five days, so only half of women will deliver by their "due date." A recent study, compiled by Australian researchers, tracked the labors and deliveries of 28,000 women—some of whom went into spontaneous labor, while others got induced for either medical or non-medical reasons. It documented a significant percentage increase in both C-section deliveries (67% increased risk), and NICU care (64%), for women and their babies who undergo non-medically necessitated inductions.

The rate of such inductions has more than doubled over the past 20 years, but some hospitals across the U.S. have recently implemented policies refusing women the option to be induced before they reach 39 weeks gestation. This trend is due in large part to studies like the Australian one, and others that indicate significant brain development taking place in babies through the 38th week of gestation. The Australian study also revealed that women giving birth after the 38th week run the lowest risk of labor complications, and women whose babies remain in utero through 41 weeks end up requiring fewer epidurals than those who deliver earlier.

Once labor begins, access to continuous labor support, such as that of a doula, has been demonstrated to reduce cesareans by 28%! Doulas do not replace doctors or midwives. They are an addition to the birth team, specializing in providing physical and emotional support to the mother. Women who use a doula are less likely to request pain medicine and more likely to report satisfaction with their birth experience. Dr. John Kennell, a physician who documented the earliest research on the benefits of doula support, said in 1998, "If a doula were a drug, it would be unethical not to use it."

LENGTH OF LABOR & "FRIEDMAN'S CURVE"

Dr. Emanuel Friedman, Professor Emeritus of Obstetrics, Gynecology, and Reproductive Biology, is world-renowned for his contributions to obstetrics, which includes a study published in 1955 describing the average amount of time it took women to dilate in labor. The study involved 500 first-time Caucasian mothers, at one hospital, who birthed at term. 70% of the moms were between the ages of 20–30. Fourteen were breech births, nine were Cesarean births, four were twin births, four were stillbirths, and 275 of them had forceps used in delivery. The babies ranged in weight from 4 lbs. 9 oz. to 10 lbs. 6 oz., with most weighing between 5 and 9 pounds. Pitocin was used to induce or augment labor in 69 people. "Twilight sleep" was a common practice back then, so 117 of the women were lightly sedated, 210 moderately sedated, and 154 deeply sedated with Demerol and scopolamine. So 96% of the women in the study were sedated with drugs!

The average length of time it took these first-time mothers to get from zero to four cm was a little over eight hours. At four centimeters dilation, the labors sped up, and they then dilated an average of 3 centimeters an hour until reaching 9 centimeters. Then the labor slowed again. The average amount of time to get from 4cm to 10cm was five hours. The average length of the pushing stage was one hour. Although the study gave doctors a way to "chart" labor, the women were sedated, and more than half of them had the babies pulled out with forceps.

Some obstetric doctors and students still use Friedman's graph as the parameter for intervening in a normal labor if it deviates from the curve. But applying a graph to all labors, which have infinite manifestations, is limiting and does not consider many factors, the primary one being that mothers are not sedated these days!

A 2010 study found that "...the rate of cervical dilation accelerated after 6 cm and progress from 4 to 6 cm was far slower than previously described. Allowing labor to continue for a longer period before 6 centimeters of cervical dilation may reduce the rate of intrapartum and subsequent repeat cesarean deliveries in the United States." (Contemporary Patterns of

Spontaneous Labor With Normal Neonatal Outcomes, *Obstetrics & Gynecology*, Zhang, Landy, et. al, 2010 Dec) A total of 62,415 mothers were selected who had a singleton term gestation, spontaneous onset of labor, vertex presentation, vaginal delivery, and a normal perinatal outcome. The average rate of dilation was 1.2 centimeters per hour, which is considered slow by Friedman's Curve. Expecting all mothers to dilate at a certain rate, at a fast pace, when their body may need more time, will often lead to a diagnosis called "Failure to Progress."

"FAILURE TO PROGRESS" AKA "LABOR ARREST"

"Failure to Progress" is a term generally used to describe a labor that has continued beyond 20 hours for first-time mothers or beyond 14 hours for a mother who has birthed before. It is also used when a laboring mother is dilating less than 1–2cm per hour during active labor. Failure to progress is the leading reason for prescribed C-section births, and is a widely used term for any labor not happening in a care provider's expected time frame.

A 2014 document titled "Safe Prevention of the Primary Cesarean Delivery," produced by the joint efforts of the ACOG and the SMFM, states, "The Consortium on Safe Labor data do not directly address an optimal duration for the diagnosis of active phase protraction or labor arrest, but do suggest that neither should be diagnosed before 6 cm of dilation. Because they are contemporary and robust, it seems that the Consortium on Safe Labor data, rather than the standards proposed by Friedman, should inform evidence-based labor management."

In other words, a labor taking longer than expected is not an indication for a C-section. This is a reason why informed consent is vitally important with regards to C-section birth. Indications for a C-section can be situations such as fetal distress (which can occur due to an induction or augmentation of labor), maternal exhaustion, concerns about blood pressure, and rare true cases of cephalopelvic disproportion (baby not fitting through the pelvis). If the mother and baby have healthy vital signs, there is no reason to opt for (or agree to) a C-section, simply because the clock is ticking faster than dilation.

POSSIBLE REASONS A LABOR MAY BE CONSIDERED A "FAILURE TO PROGRESS":

- Labor is induced prematurely, without medical necessity
- Interventions are used during birth
- Less than optimal prenatal nutrition
- Restricting movement during labor
- Uncomfortable laboring environment
- Lack of food and hydration for the mother during labor
- Constant interruption/stressing/pressuring/fear-mongering of mother

STAY LOW RISK

A mother can exert the most control over the outcome of pregnancy, her health, and the health of the baby by staying low-risk. Beginning pregnancy at a healthy weight and maintaining it throughout by eating a diet high in plant protein, a variety of fresh fruits and vegetables, avoiding added sugars and excessive carbohydrates could help prevent premature labor and birth, gestational diabetes, and other serious problems that would place a mother in the high-risk category.

Keeping a pregnancy low-risk also requires the participation of a health-care provider, and when it comes to preventing a cesarean, choosing a supportive provider can be the critical factor. A pregnant woman can interview healthcare providers and ask questions about their philosophy on birth, their current C-section rate, and the C-section rate of the facility where they deliver. There is no requirement to give birth with the provider who was overseeing gynecological care before pregnancy. Whether a woman chooses a doctor or midwife, home birth, birth center, or hospital birth, the important factor is discussing the birth plan and knowing the reasons when a cesarean might be vital. Having these conversations in advance provides the mother the option to change providers, and ultimately gives peace of mind in the case that a cesarean becomes medically necessary.

Women who give birth with midwives have a significantly lower incidence of cesarean.

VAGINAL BIRTH AFTER CESAREAN

Of particular concern is what having one C-section means for future pregnancies. The risk of cesarean surgery increases with each cesarean. Despite an increasing body of evidence that vaginal birth after cesarean is the safest option for most women, many hospitals or doctors refuse to offer/attend them. They will require women who have had one Cesarean to deliver all future children via cesarean. In 2010, the American College of Obstetrics and Gynecology announced that Vaginal Birth After Cesarean (also known as VBAC "vee-back") is the safe, appropriate, and recommended option for most women. But based on 2014 data, 90% of women who have a cesarean deliver all subsequent children by cesarean. The majority of women who attempt VBACs are successful, yet 40% of hospitals in the United States have banned VBACs in the interest of preventing lawsuits. The bans are based on outdated information, which fails to recognize the safety of vaginal birth after cesarean.

Delivery via VBAC avoids major abdominal surgery, lowers a woman's risk of hemorrhage and infection, and shortens postpartum recovery. VBAC can also help women avoid the possible future risks related to having multiple cesareans, such as hysterectomy, bowel and bladder injury, transfusion, infection, and abnormal placenta conditions, including placenta accreta and placenta previa. Placenta accreta is the clinical condition when part of the placenta or the entire placenta invades and is inseparable from the uterine wall. Placenta previa occurs when the placenta partially or completely covers the opening in the mother's cervix—the lower end of the uterus that connects to the top of the vagina. Placenta previa can cause severe bleeding before or during delivery.

Women who deliver via C-section often have a difficult time establishing breastfeeding, and babies born via C-section have a higher rate of asthma and allergies throughout their lives, which is believed to be because they are not exposed to their mother's bacteria during the birth process. Given this understanding of the benefits of vaginal birth over cesarean for most moms and babies, there is a growing movement in the field of women's health to make VBACs more accessible. (See VBAC Chapter)

RISKS AND COMPLIATIONS OF A CESAREAN SECTION

These days, many people (including some OBGYNs) consider an elective C-section a safe way of birth for babies, perhaps even safer than vaginal birth. It is not safer. Risks and complications of a C-section fall into two categories: problems experienced by the mother, and problems experienced by the baby. The most significant risk for mothers is an increased risk of death (5x more than vaginal).

CESAREAN RISKS FOR MOTHERS

Cesarean involves major abdominal surgery and increases the risk of maternal death by about four times in emergency situations and about three times during elective surgery on a healthy mother and baby. The major causes of death in these cases are infection, blood clots, and anesthetic accidents.

- Post-cesarean infections are also common. One study showed that 20 to 40 percent of women have post-cesarean complications, including infections of the uterus, wound, or urinary tract.
- Twice as likely to have severe complications and five times more likely to require antibiotics after birth.
- Another study found a three times higher risk for severe complications such as significant infection, hysterectomy, or cardiac arrest.
- Although cesareans are often portrayed as being less likely to produce pelvic floor dysfunction than vaginal birth, large population studies have demonstrated that this is not the case over the long term.

There are also psychosocial risks above and beyond the physical dangers. For example, when compared with women who give birth vaginally, women who receive a cesarean section are:

- Less satisfied with their birth experience
- More likely to be re-hospitalized
- Less confident with their babies
- Less likely to breastfeed
- More fatigued, even up to four years later

Mothers will continue to experience the effects of cesareans throughout her childbearing years. Mothers who are less satisfied with the birth experience, and felt coerced or manipulated into having a cesarean, will likely be more inclined to postpartum depression. Studies also show reduced fertility following a cesarean and higher levels of fear about giving birth. A previous cesarean may double the risk of a breech baby in subsequent pregnancies and increase the risk of uterine rupture.

CESAREAN RISKS FOR BABIES

Complications for even low-risk, healthy babies may include:

- Increased risk of respiratory compromise, low blood sugar, and poor temperature regulation.
- Slower neurological adaptation after birth.
- Differences in levels of hormones regulating calcium metabolism, renin-angiotensin, progesterone, creatine kinase, dopamine, nitric oxide synthesis, thyroid hormones, and liver enzymes.
- Depressed immune function, including poor function of neutrophils, natural killer cells, and lymphocytes (all cells that fight infection).
- Increased risk of oxidative stress.
- Cesarean delivery, as well as the drugs and antibiotics given for the surgery, affect a baby's microbiome—the microorganisms associated with its skin, mouth, nose, and gut.

෴

The alteration of the gut flora is a most significant and lasting risk for babies. Studies have consistently shown that cesarean babies have altered fecal microbiota when compared with vaginally born babies, which can persist for at least six months and possibly for life.

Among other things, the gut flora promotes normal gastrointestinal function, provides protection from infection, regulates metabolism, and comprises more than 75% of our immune system. Dysregulated gut flora has been linked to diseases such as autism and depression to autoimmune conditions like Hashimoto's, inflammatory bowel disease, and Type 1 Diabetes. Babies born via cesarean may have increased susceptibility to gut infections, asthma, allergies, and autoimmune disorders later in life. The marked changes in gut flora in cesarean babies are not significantly affected by the method of feeding (*i.e.,* breastfeeding vs. formula) afterward, which means that breastfeeding after cesarean section can't compensate for the alterations in gut flora experienced with that type of delivery.

If a mother does have a cesarean operation for any reason, it is recommended she use a high-quality infant probiotic to help populate the baby's gut with beneficial flora. (Note: there is a brand called Therbiotic Infant, from Klaire labs. They suggest starting with 1/4 tsp., which may be too much at first. Try lightly dusting the nipple with the powder once or twice a day before feedings. If you notice diarrhea, especially with green flecks or tint, decrease the dose.)

There is accumulating evidence that intestinal bacteria play an important role in the postnatal development of the immune system.

HOW TO AVOID A CESAREAN IF BABY IS BREECH?

The word breech refers to the position of the baby when the baby presents with the feet or buttocks toward the birth canal instead of head first, which is the usual and safest position. Breech is a variation of normal human birth that occurs in 3–4% of births, and vaginal delivery of a breech baby has become a bit of a lost "art." There was a time when, based on a study (Term Breech Trial), which has long since been debated, it was thought that all breech babies should be born by cesarean. After that, many practitioners stopped practicing and learning how to attend breech births, and it has become less and less common. Breech presentation is common in the middle of a pregnancy, but most babies turn themselves before 37 weeks. By 37 weeks gestation, less than 5% of babies remain in a breech position, but those who do are nearly universally birthed via C-section.

When a baby is breech after 37 weeks, there are several options a woman can pursue to encourage a baby to turn head down. There is an online resource called Spinningbabies.com. On this site, expert Gail Tully details dozens of exercises a woman can do in her own home that encourage the baby to turn on its own. The website includes instructions and videos, as well as research on how and why the techniques work.

Another option to turn a breech baby is a procedure known as an external cephalic version. In an external version, a midwife or doctor physically turns the baby from the outside, by placing her or his hands on the mother's abdomen and applying firm pressure, encouraging the baby to move into a head-down birthing position. There is a risk that this procedure will induce labor, so it is done with caution and usually in or near a hospital.

The spinning babies techniques are subtle, and an external version is a fairly invasive medical procedure, so moms seeking a moderate option when it comes to turning a breech baby may choose what is called the Webster Technique. The Webster Technique is a specific sacral adjustment performed by a trained/skilled chiropractor to help facilitate the mother's pelvic alignment and nerve system function. It may not work immediately, so give the baby some time to turn.

If the baby doesn't turn, the mother has the option to birth her baby breech. A key factor to know about breech birth is that it is prone to stop-and-start labors. Because the baby's buttocks is not putting the same pressure on the cervix as a hard head does, occasionally, you will get dramatic stopping and starting of the process. Because of this, emphasize all of the things that promote a smooth physiologic birth in any fetal position. Make sure the mother stays well nourished and supported, and minimize disruptions that may cause birth to stall. There is a saying, "Hands off the breech!" which means few or no vaginal exams, avoiding intervention, and not touching the baby at all for the birth of the buttocks and legs.

If the baby is lying in a transverse position (there is still a chance they will turn during labor), or the head is tilted, etc. "The Labor Progress Handbook" by Penny Simkin is a fantastic resource that has many suggestions in the case of malposition.

Each of us can play a role in making the healthcare system more accepting to pregnant women by being educated on these topics and advocating for change when the policies are not evidence based.

INTERNATIONAL CESAREAN AWARENESS NETWORK (ICAN)

(ICAN) is a nonprofit organization whose mission is to improve maternal-child health by preventing unnecessary cesareans through education, providing support for cesarean recovery, and promoting vaginal birth after cesarean. Their website states:

> "At ICAN – we support families as they work to advocate for themselves. With cesarean rates at all time highs – we as women must now assume more responsibility for our own births. As an organization, ICAN also advocates on behalf of the families in our communities – having critical conversations with international and regional organizations, researchers, policymakers, administrators, and birth professionals – making sure that our voices are heard, and that key decision makers can better understand the often complicated issues surrounding cesarean and VBAC."

IF EMERGENCY CESAREAN IS NECESSARY ASK FOR WHAT YOU WANT

- ☐ Request that the mother walk to the operating room, if able to do so
- ☐ Ask (or demand) that the partner accompanies the mother to the room, and for the operation preparation
- ☐ Request that the mother's arms are not strapped down
- ☐ Request that the lights be dimmed as much as possible
- ☐ Request an epidural or spinal block; avoiding general anesthesia at all costs, except for emergencies
- ☐ Request that anesthesiologists do not automatically give extra drugs, so that the mother can be fully present
- ☐ If the mother has a heart monitoring device or baby monitoring devices, they can be placed in areas that don't infringe her ability to see, hold or breastfeed baby
- ☐ Ask that the doctors be extra gentle in handling the baby
- ☐ Mother can watch the baby lifted from her belly through a clear drape

- ☐ Ask to place baby skin to skin on the mother's bare chest while she is being sutured
- ☐ If the mother cannot be conscious, the partner can hold the baby skin-to-skin immediately after birth
- ☐ Ask for the uterus to be closed with a double layer of sutures
- ☐ Baby can breastfeed immediately while in the operating room
- ☐ Request prolonged cord clamping and cutting until it stops pulsing/has turned white (reminders usually necessary)
- ☐ Request that the placenta be saved and frozen until leaving the hospital, if desired
- ☐ Play soothing music of your choice in the operating room
- ☐ Ask doctors and nurses to refrain from "shop talk" (*i.e.,* doctors should not converse about scars, incisions, football, weekend plans, lunch, etc.)
- ☐ Ask the doctor for a vaginal swab to give baby the best microbiome
- ☐ Mother can hold the baby while being wheeled to post-op and recovery unit
- ☐ Ask to delay all post-birth procedures such as cleaning and weighing the baby, until parents are ready and say so
- ☐ Ask that a friend, doula, or grandparent are permitted inside for support, and to photograph or videotape the birth so the parents can concentrate on bonding

NECESSSARY EMERGENCY CESAREANS

As mentioned before, C-sections can be life-saving operations for the child, mother, or both. Mothers have been in situations where they labored for days and reached point of exhaustion, or the baby was indeed stuck, or there was a uterine rupture, or there were deformities/abnormalities of the baby's body, or birth defects of the baby, an umbilical cord prolapse, etc., and it was imperative that the baby be removed from her body.

The statement often said to her following the birth is, "But you have a healthy baby." Indeed a healthy baby is the desired outcome for all parents. But for a mother, the desired outcome for her birth may also have been a vaginal birth, and she may thereby feel devastated. This mother is delicate and needs proper support and a lot of love. She will feel a flood of emotions, her body will be recovering, and she will need someone to listen to her and comfort her, as she reconciles her experience.

A mother who has had a cesarean is no less of a mother and has still nourished, grown, and birthed a child with her miraculous body.

"Untitled"

"And after three days he cried Mama. Mama, I cannot come to you. Mama, I am so tired. Mama, please reach in, please send help. Mama, I cannot finish the journey alone. And in the wee hours of the third day, she lay down her ego, she lay down her pride, she poured her tears on the earth. And she cut a hole in her own flesh to do what all mothers do-that which must be done. She rent her dreams to make a way, and she brought her sweet baby home."

– Ann, 2011, Midwestern US (from "Homebirth Cesarean")

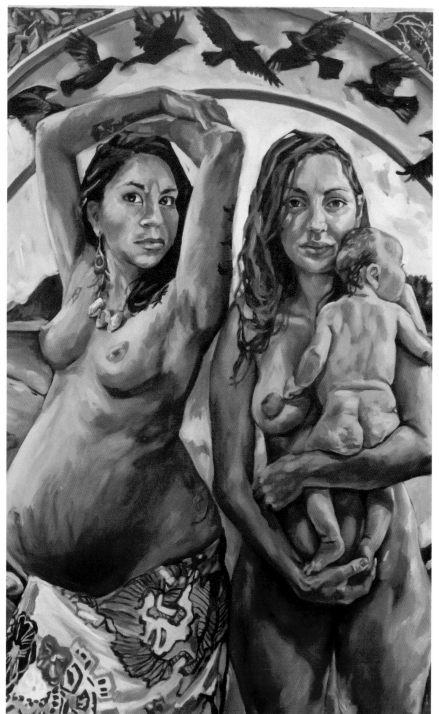

CHAPTER 13:
OBSTETRIC VIOLENCE

"Although the popularly desired outcome is 'healthy mother, healthy baby,' I think there is room in that equation for 'happy, non-traumatized, empowered and elated mother and baby.'"
- MIDWIFERY TODAY

"The effort to separate the physical experience of childbirth from the mental, emotional and spiritual aspects of this event has served to disempower and violate women."
- MARY HUCKLOS HAMPTON

"Birth should not be a time in a woman's life when she has to FIGHT for anything."
- CARLA HARTLEY

MY FATHER, WHO IS an outstanding doctor, after reading this chapter, remarked that it just couldn't be true. Because it is an appalling reality that those who are chosen to care for another would create such suffering. I know it is true, I told him, because I have read many stories that are not fabrications. I have had mothers at parks relay their traumatic birth to me. I have seen it with my own two eyes—a mother trying to give birth with another woman's hands up inside of her, "helping to stretch her," while the mother is saying it doesn't feel good. The content in this chapter is real—both the subtle violence and the overt. It is happening all over.

Birthing mothers are regularly subject to traumatic, dehumanizing care and violations of their human rights. The term "obstetric violence," as it appears in the Organic Law on the Right of Women to Be Free from Violence, was enacted in Venezuela on March 16, 2007. The law defines obstetric violence as:

"The appropriation of the body and reproductive processes of women by health personnel, which is expressed as dehumanized treatment, an abuse of medication, and to convert the natural processes into pathological ones, bringing with it loss of autonomy and the ability to decide freely about their bodies and sexuality, negatively impacting the quality of life of women."

The phrase "the appropriation of the body and reproductive processes of women by health personnel" is, according to Dr. Pérez D'Gregorio, "contrary to good obstetric practice, whereby medication should only be used when it is indicated, the natural processes should be respected, and instrumental or surgical procedures should be performed only when the indication follows evidence-based medicine."

Obstetric violence is institutional violence, violence against women, and violation of human rights. It can occur during pregnancy, at childbirth, and in the post partum period. It occurs both in public and private medical practices. Obstetric violence is also manifested by discrimination based on race, ethnic, or economic background, as well as age, body type, HIV status, and gender non-conformity, among other factors. It is an overlooked and normalized type of violence against women, which complicates the design of public policies to prevent and eradicate it.

For too many women, pregnancy is a period associated with suffering, humiliation, ill health, and even death. Obstetric violence may be manifested through denial of treatment during childbirth, disregard of a woman's needs and pain, and verbal humiliation. It may also be manifested through forced and coerced medical interventions, invasive practices, and unnecessary use of medications. Women may suffer dehumanizing or rude treatment and even detention in facilities for failure to pay.

Every woman has the right to access skilled and high-quality care during childbirth. The State is responsible for institutional violence when women are denied access to health care, treated inhumanely, forced, or coerced into unnecessary medical procedures or when denied the right to choose them.

EXAMPLES OF OBSTETRIC VIOLENCE

- Procedure without consent (vaginal exam, rupture of membranes, medication administration, etc.) or coercing her to give consent
- Forced operation (refusal of a VBAC or a vaginal breech birth)
- Demeaning communication (*e.g.,* "You don't know what you're talking about" "Who's the professional here?" "I have doctor's orders")
- Refusal to disclose options (*i.e.,* a second opinion, alternate provider, alternate birth locations)
- Physical violence during labor and delivery, including slapping, pushing on the abdomen to force the baby out, and excessive force on the fetus
- Lack of informed consent
- Misinformation about delivery options and methods
- Disrespect for non-medical delivery methods such as water births, use of a doula, and home delivery
- Belittling mother's choices
- Lack of confidentiality
- Fear mongering of the laboring mother
- Forced sterilization
- Pressure mother to get an epidural after she's declined multiple times
- Untimely and ineffective attention of obstetric emergencies
- Forcing the woman to birth in a supine position, with legs raised, when the necessary means to perform a vertical delivery are available
- Impeding the early attachment of the child with his/her mother without a medical cause, thus preventing the early attachment and blocking the possibility of holding, nursing, or breast-feeding immediately after birth. Medical staff will spend these crucial moments weighing baby, putting on bracelets, etc., saying, "Oh, it will just be five minutes."
- Altering the natural process of low-risk delivery by using acceleration techniques, without obtaining voluntary, expressed and informed consent of the woman, as well as increasing drug dosage without consent
- Performing delivery via cesarean section, when natural childbirth is possible, without obtaining voluntary, expressed, and informed consent from the woman

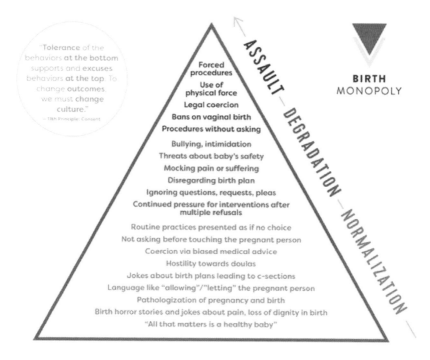

"Tolerance of the behaviors at the bottom supports and excuses behaviors at the top. To change outcomes, we must change culture."

– 18th Principle: Consent

ASSAULT — DEGRADATION — NORMALIZATION

BIRTH MONOPOLY

Forced procedures
Use of physical force
Legal coercion
Bans on vaginal birth
Procedures without asking

Bullying, intimidation
Threats about baby's safety
Mocking pain or suffering
Disregarding birth plan
Ignoring questions, requests, pleas
Continued pressure for interventions after multiple refusals

Routine practices presented as if no choice
Not asking before touching the pregnant person
Coercion via biased medical advice
Hostility towards doulas
Jokes about birth plans leading to c-sections
Language like "allowing"/"letting" the pregnant person
Pathologization of pregnancy and birth
Birth horror stories and jokes about pain, loss of dignity in birth
"All that matters is a healthy baby"

PHYSICAL ABUSE

Physical abuse of a birthing woman can include procedures without consent but can also take the form of patient neglect. One woman shared that she was left to bleed for four hours following the birth of her fourth baby. She was found when a new midwife came on duty in the hospital and was rushed to surgery to repair a 6.5-cm tear in her cervix. The previous midwife on duty had ignored her concerns about the bleeding.

VERBAL ABUSE

Verbal obstetric violence occurs when a care provider insults, ridicules, yells at or threatens a pregnant, laboring, or postpartum woman. Things like, "Why did you take off your panties?" "I need you to be delivered by now." "At this point, we're either fishin' or cuttin' the bait." "You aren't allowed to." Women are ridiculed by medical staff for refusing pain relief: "You don't need to be a superhero," or for verbalizing through contractions: "Be quiet—you sound ridiculous!" It's also fairly common for women to be threatened with physical violence: "If you show up here in labor, we will simply take you straight for a cesarean," is commonly said to women planning a VBAC at non-supportive hospitals.

EMOTIONAL ABUSE

Pregnant women are especially at risk of emotional abuse. With all the hormones, doubts, fears, and concerns, it's easy to scare a pregnant woman. Merely suggesting that a mother doesn't care about her baby is a form of abuse that is VERY prevalent. Here are some actual quotes from care providers encountered during pregnancy that indeed constitute emotional abuse:

"You must get induced. Your risk of stillbirth is increasing, and it would be very traumatic for the staff if your baby died."
"I have been unable to sleep all week as I'm scared your baby will die."
"You obviously want a vaginal birth more than a live baby."

There was no indication that these mothers were experiencing anything other than a healthy pregnancy with a healthy baby. Yet these care providers felt the need to bully the mothers into consenting to inductions. As Ina May Gaskin has stated, "It is very easy, even profitable, to scare pregnant women. But it's not nice, so we shouldn't do it."

ECONOMIC ABUSE

If a woman, particularly one who is deemed by the hospital to be "high risk," wishes to access evidence-based, woman-centered care from a known midwife (shown time and again to improve outcomes for mothers and babies), she must be able to pay from $2000–$4000 for an independent midwife to attend her at home. If she doesn't have the money, she is then unable to access the care of her choice and must instead receive the "standard care" covered by her insurance plan. Many women find that they can't afford the care that they prefer or feel will be best for them. By no means am I suggesting that independent midwives should not charge appropriately for their services, they deserve much more actually. It must be recognized that a patriarchal system decides who can attend a woman through financial control.

There is also a level of economic abuse from private obstetricians. I hear from many women who are told by their private OBGYN that they will not discuss birth plans until late in the pregnancy, even telling some mothers that they will not say until 38 weeks whether or not they will support a VBAC. By this stage, the woman has paid a large amount of non-refundable fees to the obstetrician. Due to this fact, many women feel unable or unwilling so late in the pregnancy to switch to a supportive care provider if their current one proves to be unsupportive.

SEXUAL ABUSE

It is important to remember that it is a woman's sexual organs that are generally subject to abuse. In any other setting, if someone puts their hand or instruments inside a woman's vagina when she has asked them not to, or are telling them (or screaming) "NO," that constitutes rape. Yet it is not considered so if it happens in a hospital. In fact, it is downplayed as "for the good of the baby" or "necessary." Cervical exams are an example of routine care accepted as normal.

In labor, a cervical exam is a way to check how dilated a mother is upon admittance to the hospital or birthing center. Often, women are offered cervical checks towards the end of pregnancy to see where they are. It is important to note the following about cervical exams: there is a lack of evidence to support them, they are not the only way to decide if labor is active, they are not the only way to assess progress, they are not always accurate, and they cannot predict the future. They can also reverse dilation, due to the mother being interrupted, feeling threatened, invaded, or stressed (often because of the frequent exams and the commentary about her progress of dilation. There is also a risk of infection and premature rupture of membranes (PROM). In an undisturbed labor, a mother can just be observed for the signs of progress and dilation, and the urges to push when her body is ready.

The idea that "doctor knows best" is what can lead mothers to agreeing (or not agreeing) to things like cervical exams in labor. The same approach that "doctor knows best" can lead to their performing acts on the mother that violate her psyche and/or body. When the laboring mother feels safe and is trusted to know her body, and it's functions, the outcomes are more optimal. The mother is the one experiencing the labor, and no one cares about the baby's well being more than the mother (of course, there are rare cases of exception here).

EXPOSING THE SILENCE PROJECT

As many as 1/3 of American women say that the birth of their child was traumatic. Activist Cristen Pascucci and doula/photographer Lindsay Askins drove across America for two months in 2015, photographing and interviewing women who have experienced and witnessed traumatic births and obstetric violence, asking them:

"What was traumatic about your baby's birth?"

"What happened if you tried to tell people about it?"

"How are you taking your power back?"

Their website (Exposing the Silence Project.com) states:

> "It's time to meet these women and document their stories. It's time for women to feel validated in their feelings and experiences. It's time for the general public to be aware that obstetric violence is a very real and serious issue in the United States. It's time for women to feel confident in speaking out about their trauma during childbirth. It's time for the legal system to take these cases seriously and consider them viable in a court of law. It's time for the maternity care system to drastically change the way pregnant and birthing women are perceived and treated."

⌇

The next time you hear a friend relay a story where she feels that she was violated, bullied, disempowered, coerced, or assaulted, let her know that what she experienced has a name. Many women have found that being able to put a name to their experiences is a part of being able to commence her healing journey. Let her know that she is not crazy, and she is not alone. Exposing The Silence Project's website has extensive stories from mothers about obstetric violence and birth trauma. These are personal accounts based on first-hand experience and can be rather unsettling.

Black women are three to four times more likely to experience a pregnancy-related death than white women.

HUMAN RIGHTS

> "Birth is a feminist issue and a human rights crisis. My mission is to flip the system upside down so that women and birthing people are on top." – Cristen Pascucci

After the birth of her son in 2011, Cristen Pascucci left a career in public affairs to study American maternity care and women's rights within it. Cristen is the inspiring founder of Birth Monopoly, co-creator of the Exposing the Silence Project, and former vice president of the national consumer advocacy organization Improving Birth. She has ran an emergency hotline for women facing threats to their legal rights in childbirth, created a viral consumer campaign to "Break the Silence" on trauma and abuse in childbirth, and helped put the maternity care crisis in national media. She is a leading voice for women giving birth, speaking and consulting around the country on issues related to birth rights and options, and working on a documentary about the mistreatment of birthing women titled "Mother: May I."

Mothers are human beings, and it is a fundamental human right to determine the circumstances of where, how, and with whom you give birth. There is tremendous interference with this right in the form of overly restrictive midwifery regulation, state regulations, hospital policies, and hospitals and doctors defending themselves in courtrooms all over the country claiming the authority to override a woman's decisions at their discretion.

Birth Monopoly is an extensive online resource and archive for the topic of human rights in childbirth and obstetric violence. You will find classes like, "Know Your Rights: Legal and Human Rights in Childbirth for Birth Professionals and Advocates," articles on obstetric violence, and stories from women all over the world. The Podcast *Birth Allowed Radio* has episodes such as a doula's "How to Advocate Without Getting Kicked Out of The Room," an assaulted mother's "My Injury is Forever and a Lifetime," and a lawyer's "The Problem with Implied Consent." Cristen's article, "You're Not Allowed to Not Allow Me" addresses, in her words, the outdated, sexist protocols about how we are "allowed" to give birth—how much time we're 'allowed'— what position we're 'allowed' to be in—whether or not we're 'allowed' to walk around or eat or drink- whether or not we are 'allowed' to say 'NO!' when it comes to our bodies, our babies, our own births-hospitals 'not allowing' women to birth a baby out of their own vaginas if they've had a previous Cesarean—and those same hospitals lobby in the statehouse to make sure those women aren't 'allowed' to have the right at home, either." I have included two of her articles, with her permission, below.

YOU'RE NOT ALLOWED TO NOT ALLOW ME
by Cristen Pascucci, June 17, 2014

> "In law and ethics, it is the patient who chooses to allow the provider to do something, not the other way around."

For most women, pregnancy and childbirth are one of the few times we let other adults tell us what we are "allowed" and "not allowed" to do with our own bodies. It's time to change our language around this to reflect the legal and ethical reality that it is the patient who chooses to allow the provider to do something—not the other way around—and to eliminate **a word that has no place between true partners in care**.

We hear the word "allow" used regularly, by well-meaning care providers and family members, and by pregnant women themselves. During my own pregnancy, I was told I **"may or may not be allowed" to hold my baby** immediately after he was born, depending on what hospital staff was on shift. It struck me as so odd that I might be in the position of asking to hold my own precious baby, especially when I'd chosen to hire these care providers. Who was allowing whom here?

Most recently, it has been all over the media following the March 2014 release of guidelines for lowering the primary Cesarean rate from the American College of Obstetricians and Gynecologists (ACOG) and the Society for Maternal-Fetal Medicine:

"Women with low-risk pregnancies should be *allowed* to spend more time in labor, to reduce the risk of having an unnecessary C-section, the nation's obstetricians say." (NPR.org)

OR "That may mean that we *allow* a patient to labor longer, to push for a longer amount of time, and to *allow* patients to take more time through the natural process." (CBS News Philadelphia)

For women giving birth in the American maternity system, these guide-lines are welcome, but they are no magic bullet. Medical practices take years and even decades to change, and while that happens, **what assurances do women have** about the care they are receiving *today*? Is it ethical to hold women to what an individual provider will "allow," with the full knowledge that not all providers are practicing to the standards science show is best for moms and babies?

These are not rhetorical questions. In the U.S., outdated, non-evidence-based practice is routine and accepted; Cesarean section rates vary ten-fold among U.S. hospitals; and those rates vary fifteen-fold among the low-risk population. Over 40% of hospitals defy national health policy by "not allow-ing" vaginal birth after Cesarean, to the detriment of hundreds of thousands of mothers and babies. The United States is the only developed country in the world with a RISING maternal mortality rate. One factor in that rise is our overuse of surgery for childbirth. **We simply cannot operate on the assumption that the surgeries women are receiving are always in their best interests, or that of their babies.**

But it's about more than just a stand-alone decision around whether to do a Cesarean. There's a sequence of events leading up to that possibility, and **many women have been relieved of their decision-making** well before that time. When women have been given messages all along that they are not the authority in their own childbirth, it's easy for a care provider to make a unilateral decision about surgery. What woman, who has experienced nine months of language like "we can't let you" and "you're not allowed" is going to suddenly have the wherewithal to refuse an unnecessary surgery—or to even know **she has the right to do so?**

The truth is that women, like all other U.S. citizens, have the right to make decisions about their bodies based on informed consent—a legal, ethical standard which requires the provider to convey all of the information around a suggested procedure or course of treatment, and the person receiving the procedure or treatments gets to decide whether or not to take that advice. ACOG states clearly about informed consent in maternity care: "The freedom to accept or refuse recommended medical treatment has legal as well as ethical foundations. . . . In the obstetric setting, recognize that a competent pregnant woman is the appropriate decision maker for the fetus that she is carrying"

(ACOG Committee on Ethics Committee Opinion No. 390 *Ethical Decision Making in Obstetrics and Gynecology;* Dec 2007, reaffirmed 2013).

This stands in stark contrast to women being told they are "not allowed" to decline potentially harmful interventions like continuous electronic monitoring in a low-risk pregnancy, or to make an informed decision for a vaginal birth rather than a surgical one—or even to eat, drink, or go to the bathroom in labor.

At its heart, this language is about **a lack of respect**. It's how we speak to children, not competent adults. It's a sloppy way of skipping meaningful and necessary conversations about what should be a common goal for both mother and provider: a healthy, happy birth.

It's also a reinforcement of deep cultural beliefs about women as passive objects, not full owners of their bodies nor representatives of their babies, and having lesser decision-making capacity than those they've hired to support them. These ideas will take time to change. But birth is a great place to start.

Words have power, and **we can take back that power** in simple ways:

- Don't stay silent when you hear this kind of language in casual conversation. Say something—even if it's just a little something. Don't let it go unnoticed.
- Be gentle while you are being firm. Remember that most people are just repeating something common and accepted, and they probably haven't thought much about it. Make it your goal to inform, not convince.
- Choose to give your business to providers who use respectful language. If you're hearing this language during pregnancy, you can be pretty sure you're going to hear it during childbirth—and that can be a problem. You can't act like a mother when you're being treated like a child.
- Partners, stand up for your loved ones. When she is vulnerable, be her voice. There is no one better positioned to be a vocal advocate for her and her baby.

Today, American women are gambling with their bodies when they give birth, with a one in three average Cesarean rate in facilities where practices vary widely, even among individual providers. And **we are tying women's hands when we continue to reinforce this dysfunction** by using words like "allow" to describe an outdated dynamic that doesn't recognize us as competent, rights-bearing adults.

The legal authority in childbirth lies with the woman giving birth, not the providers of care. Yes, they are a team, but of the two, it is the woman who truly bears the rights and the risks of childbirth. Our words should reflect that reality.

BEING ADMITTED TO THE HOSPITAL OR SIGNING CONSENT FORMS IS NOT "IMPLIED CONSENT"

by Cristen Pascucci, September 18, 2017

Even in 2017, women's consent rights in childbirth are disturbingly unclear to the professionals and institutions delivering their medical care. One aspect is the idea of "implied consent"—a concept mischaracterized by hospitals to a number of women who have contacted me, and sometimes used to justify violations of their dignity and rights.

Specifically, when these women have complained to their hospitals about receiving one or more non-consented or forced procedures in birth, they were told that their explicit consent was not necessary because they had:

1. agreed to be admitted to the hospital or
2. signed blanket consent forms giving medical staff permission to treat them

Sometimes these hospitals refer to this, erroneously, as "implied consent." The idea is that once the women were admitted or signed those forms, they should no longer have had the expectation that the care team must obtain consent for *each* procedure during treatment—including medication, surgical cuts, and procedures performed on and through the vagina—but, rather, expect that the care team had the authority to administer whatever treatment they chose for the duration of that patient's labor or hospital stay. Put another way, from the perspective of the hospital, these women had forfeited their rights to informed consent and refusal in order to give birth in their facilities. This belief by hospitals is wrong, legally and ethically.

First, let's take a rational look at this idea by pulling it back to all medical care—not just Labor & Delivery. We can make this comparison because patients are patients, whether they are in the emergency department or in Labor & Delivery. Patients in Labor & Delivery do not have different, or fewer, legal rights than other patients. Pregnant or not, you retain your basic legal rights. (Caveat: there are certain states where fetal personhood laws conflict with this idea and make things a little more tricky, but there is no broad, statutory law that conveys a different set of rights or restricts the rights of pregnant people in the United States.) Neither is there any law that endows obstetricians or L&D departments with special legal authority over the medical care of their patients who are pregnant.

Obstetricians and hospitals certainly have tried to claim this right in court—for example, in testimony for *Malatesta vs. Brookwood Medical Center*, or when lawyers defending the hospital in *Dray* vs. Staten Island University Hospital, et al. argued that doctors do not need to wait for a court order to "override" a woman's refusal of surgery in labor (that is, that they do not need to respect her right to due process); or when the implicated doctor in *Switzer vs. Rezvina* argued she doesn't need to respect pregnant women's decisions. Despite these claims, there is no general basis for a hospital to argue that implied consent applies in any way differently on their L&D unit or to their pregnant patients than it would to the rest of the hospital or non-pregnant patients.

With that in mind, consider the effect of the idea that admission to a hospital is "implied consent" for treatment: No patient would ever have the right to information about their medical care or the right to say "no" to it. Informed consent—the basic legal right to receive information and give or refuse permission in our medical care—cannot co-exist with this flawed definition of implied consent. The concepts contradict each other.

In fact, "implied consent" in medical care is something that is generally understood to apply to emergency situations when the person is *both* unconscious and incapable of consent (*i.e.,* a person presents at an E.R. with a gunshot wound and then passes out before he can agree to a certain course of treatment). It is a concept with very limited scope that applies to a limited range of situations—none of which are the very broad scope of *pregnancy*. Moreover, says, attorney Farah Diaz-Tello, formerly of National

Advocates for Pregnant Women and a specialist in birth law, "Implied consent *never* overrides non-consent. So if someone walked in a hospital with a baby hanging out of her vagina, she has implicitly consented to their treating her by seeking help. But the second she says 'no, stop that,' they have to stop. She hasn't consented to every possible thing ever. You might consent by seeking help, but *consent is always revocable.*"

The idea that consent is always revocable brings us to our next point: the confusion around consent forms and the power they do or do not have. I have heard pregnant women and medical professionals state that executing consent forms means "signing away your rights." In one case of a woman receiving a non-consented membrane stripping during a consented vaginal exam, she was told by a hospital representative, "When you sign the consent for care, that goes from the beginning all the way through until discharge"; in context, the hospital representative was saying that once the patient had signed a consent form at admission, they did not need her ongoing permission to administer medical procedures. This belief is also wrong, legally and ethically.

The American College of Obstetricians and Gynecologists (ACOG), says plainly:

> "Often, informed consent is confused with the consent form. In fact, informed consent is 'the willing acceptance of a medical intervention by a patient after adequate disclosure by the physician of the nature of the intervention with its risks and benefits and of the alternatives with their risks and benefits'. The consent form only documents the process and the patient decision." (From Committee on Ethics Committee Opinion #390, "Ethical Decision Making in Obstetrics and Gynecology," 2013)

ACOG is clear that the documentation of informed consent is fundamentally different from the actual process of informed consent—a process based on a constitutionally based idea that human beings own their own bodies, enshrined in a right that extends to their medical care. We should also remember that *consent forms and informed consent are primarily meant to protect the patient.* Something has gone terribly awry when hospitals use these protections *against* patients, rather than in defense of them.

Indeed, based on my extensive interactions with unhappy maternity care customers, hospitals seem to routinely respond to complaints about violations of informed consent with something along the lines of, "We're sorry for the communication problem, but your treatment was medically appropriate"— and then claim the patient didn't have the right to say no to the treatment in the first place. ACOG says otherwise:

> "Obstetrician-gynecologists are discouraged in the strongest possible terms from the use of duress, manipulation, coercion, physical force, or threats, including threats to involve the courts or child protective services, to motivate women toward a specific clinical decision…pregnancy does not lessen or limit the requirement to obtain informed consent or to honor a pregnant woman's refusal of recommended treatment." (From Committee on Ethics Committee Opinion #664, "Refusal of Medically Recommended Treatment During Pregnancy," 2016)

I can think of several women off the top of my head who had vaginal exams without their consent, or who consented to the vaginal exam but then had had an additional procedure forced on them in the course of the exam. For example, in the previously mentioned story documented in Episode 8 of *Birth Allowed Radio*, the hospital representatives claimed repeatedly to the woman that a membrane sweep (meant to induce labor) is *part of* a vaginal exam (meant to assess dilation), so she did not have a right to refuse it once she had consented to the vaginal exam. (This claim, by the way, that an assessment of cervical dilation includes a manual induction of labor, is false. These are two stand-alone procedures with separate functions.) One representative said to her: "So [the physicians] feel like, you know, their fingers are up in your vagina and you've consented to *that*, so…"

Essentially, this hospital, like other hospitals, justified a physician's actions by pinpointing the moment they claim the patient *no longer has consent rights*— the moment the medical professional assumes control of the patient's body… ostensibly at the request of the patient. That is wrong from any angle and easily fits a definition of obstetric violence as "appropriation" of the patient's body. There is no moment when a patient forfeits the rights of informed consent and refusal, short of a serious medical emergency where the patient is *unable* to consent. It is especially alarming when, as in another situation with a non-consented membrane sweep, that hospital defended its physician with an "implied consent" argument even when the woman loudly, explicitly refused the procedure after it started happening. The hospital used her own prior consent to justify the physician inflicting that humiliation and trauma on her *even as she was crying, "No!"* This is simply unjustifiable.

These are foundational legal and patients rights issues, and yet the front line of communications in many hospitals doesn't seem to have, or isn't willing to admit they have, a basic grasp of them. In fact, in both of the specific situations I've mentioned in this article, each hospital conducted an internal physician review of the patient's complaint before responding. So, it seems that neither administrations *nor the physicians* at these facilities have a working understanding of the legal and ethical obligations owed to patients for informed consent and refusal.

One hospital representative also said she'd contacted other local hospitals about their consent processes, and they agreed they did not have a consent process for stripping women's membranes in the course of a vaginal exam. It's fair to say, then, that this hospital representative's major errors about the ideas of implied consent, informed consent, and consent forms are not unique to her or the facility where she works.

All hospitals that provide maternity services should note that women are bringing lawsuits about informed consent violations in childbirth—most recently, the California case where a woman sued her doctor for medical battery following a forced, explicitly refused episiotomy. Several cases revolving around informed consent and refusal in childbirth have also been resolved in and out of court over the last year or so in Washington, Alabama, and New Jersey.

Informed consent and consent forms protect patients, but they also protect healthcare professionals. A medical professional should not be held liable for adverse outcomes resulting from a patient's informed decision about their own medical care, and documentation of a patients' refusal of treatment is a liability protection for the care providers involved. If that principle rings hollow to lawsuit-shy practitioners, there are lawyers and experts in the birth-rights movement willing to testify to it. Instead of blaming patients who have been harmed by institutional failures to respect informed consent and refusal, hospitals must look critically at what is happening in their facilities. They should have written policies and in-house educational requirements based on current, accurate interpretations of care providers' legal duties to patients, with meaningful feedback loops for patient complaints. Sometimes, this will mean hospitals need to admit they have been doing it wrong for a long time. That moment of truth is a small and necessary price for earning women's trust in the future.

∾

Prevention and Treatment of Traumatic Childbirth (PATTCh)

"If a woman experiences or perceives that she and/or her baby were in danger of injury or death to during childbirth, her birth is defined as traumatic —psychologically, physically, or both. Usually, she experiences extreme sense of helplessness, isolation, lack of care, fear, and anxiety. Traumatic childbirth occurs in as many as 25–34 per cent of all births. Approximately one-third of those women may develop Posttraumatic Stress Disorder (PTSD)."

– PATTCh website

The PATTCh board members are a group of psychotherapists, childbirth educators, doulas, researchers, and academicians who are dedicated to bringing together like-minded individuals to educate childbearing women and families and maternity care professionals; develop effective prenatal, intrapartum and postpartum care practices to prevent or reduce traumatic birth and post-birth PTSD; and identify and promote effective treatments to enhance recovery.

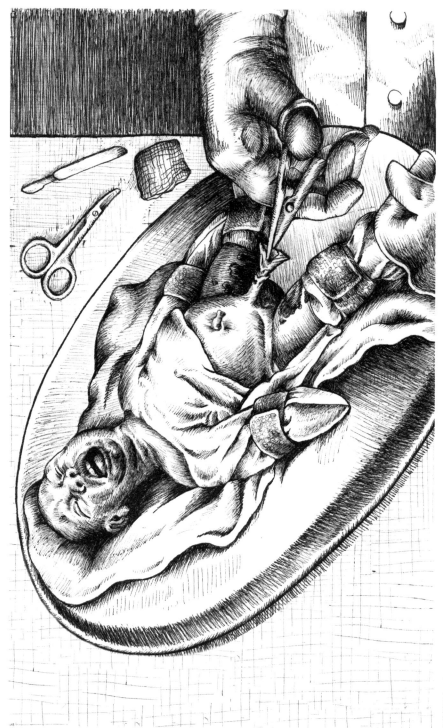

Nikki Scioscia

CHAPTER 14:
GENITAL MUTILATION

*"Circumcision is a painful, risky, unethical surgery
that deprives over a million boys each year of healthy,
functional tissue, while wasting health care dollars that
could be spent on medically necessary services."*
- INTACT AMERICA

"Please don't do this to me."
- CRIED EVERY NEWBORN BEING CUT EVER

*"How strange that excision – female circumcision, with several
languages using the same term for both kinds of mutilation
– of little girls should revolt the westerner but excite no
disapproval when it is performed on little boys. Consensus on
the point seems absolute. But ask your interlocutor to think
about the validity of this surgical procedure, which consists of
removing a healthy part of a nonconsenting child's body on
nonmedical grounds – the legal definition of... mutilation."*
- MICHEL ONFRAY
*Atheist Manifesto: The Case Against Christianity,
Judaism, and Islam*

THIS CHAPTER IS BIASED. I have a son whom I did not have cut. I consider "circumcision" a human rights issue. The content below is intended for expecting mothers and partners, with the hope that they will reconsider cutting their child's genitals if they have not already. If you have already done so to *your child* or children, please read on anyway, as there is always something to learn. Like, the average hospital cost of a circumcision nationwide is about $2,000, according to the Department of Health and Human Services. Dr. David Chamberlain tells us in *The Mind of the Newborn* that everything matters, for the fetus and the newborn remembers it all.

WHAT IS CIRCUMCISION?

The word comes from Latin circumcidere, meaning "to cut around." Circumcision is the surgical removal of the foreskin, also called prepuce, from the human penis. In the most common procedure, the foreskin is opened and then separated from the glans after inspection. The circumcision device (if used) is placed, and the foreskin removed. Topical or locally injected anesthesia is occasionally used to reduce pain and physiologic stress. The procedure is most often an elective surgery performed on neonates and children for religious and cultural reasons, or because it is the norm. This invasive procedure carries serious health risks, including infection, hemorrhage, surgical mishap, and death, as well as many ethical considerations.

Why would the foreskin be there in the first place if it weren't meant to be there? Isn't that like saying it's a mistake? Why is it considered too painful to do later in life, but somehow not as painful for a newborn, who has just left the safety and comfort of the dark womb? The exit into this realm is the most sensitive, fragile time in our life, adapting and trusting that we will be cared for and protected. When I told someone that I would not be circumcising my son, they replied, "But it's cleaner." I, in turn, asked, "What do you mean? How so?" They did not respond.

For the record, an uncircumcised penis is not dirty. There is no need to pull back the foreskin on an infant to clean beneath it. Over time, the foreskin will retract on its own, which happens at different times for different boys, but most can retract their foreskins by the time they're five years old.

NOT RECOMMENDED

Newborn male circumcision is one of the most common surgical procedures performed in the United States. Approximately 55% to 65% of all infant boys are circumcised in the U.S. each year. Circumcision is usually performed during the first ten days of a person's life, but most often within the first 48 hours, either in the hospital or, for some religious rituals, at home.

Circumcision is routinely recommended and endorsed by doctors and other health professionals, but the fact is, no professional medical association in the U.S. or anywhere in the world recommends routine circumcision as medically necessary.

An estimated one-fourth of males worldwide are circumcised. The procedure is most prevalent in the Muslim world and Israel (where it is near-universal as a religious obligation), the United States, and parts of Southeast Asia and Africa. It is relatively rare in Europe, Latin America, parts of Southern Africa and most of Asia. The origin of circumcision is not known with certainty; the oldest documented evidence comes from ancient Egypt. Various theories have been proposed of the background, including as a religious sacrifice and as a rite of passage marking a boy's entrance into adulthood. It is part of religious law in Judaism and is an established practice in Islam, Coptic Christianity, and the Ethiopian Orthodox Church.

SO WHY IS IT DONE?

People say that circumcised infants are less likely to develop urinary tract infections (UTIs), especially in the first year of life. UTIs are about ten times more common in uncircumcised males than circumcised ones. However, even with this increased risk of UTI, only 1% or fewer of uncircumcised males will ever get a UTI.

- Circumcised men also might be at lower risk for penile cancer, although the disease is rare in both circumcised and uncircumcised males.
- Penile problems such as irritation, inflammation, and infection are more common in uncircumcised males.

*None of the above subjective findings are conclusive.

In ancient days, circumcision, and more extensive mutilation of the external genitalia was carried out on defeated enemies, captives, or slaves as a sign of subjugation.

The world's major medical organizations' position ranges from considering elective neonatal and child circumcision as having no benefit and significant risks, to having a modest health benefit that outweighs small risks. No major medical organization recommends either universal circumcision for all males or banning the procedure. Ethical and legal questions regarding informed consent and human rights are all raised over child and infant circumcision.

PRIMARY REASONS PEOPLE GIVE FOR CUTTING THEIR CHILDREN:
- Religion
- Fear of child being different
- To be like his dad
- Cleanliness
- It's just what you do (normalcy)

PAIN RELIEF?

The procedure is painful. In the past, it wasn't common to provide any pain relief. But the American Academy of Pediatrics (AAP) recommends pain relief, and studies show that infants who undergo circumcision benefit from anesthesia. I'm not sure why they needed a study to show that anesthesia would help lessen the pain when cutting the tip of the penis of a newborn. Thus, most doctors now use it, but it is still a relatively new standard of care.

Two main types of local anesthetic are used to make the operation less painful for a baby:
- A topical cream (a cream put on the penis) that requires at least 20 to 40 minutes to take its full effect;
- An injectable anesthetic that requires less time to take effect and may provide a slightly longer period of numbness.

In addition to anesthesia, an acetaminophen suppository can be inserted in the baby's rectum, which can help reduce discomfort during the procedure and several hours afterward. Sometimes the newborn is given a pacifier dipped in sugar water to help reduce the stress and pain.

It usually takes between 7 to 10 days for a penis to heal. Initially, the tip will appear slightly swollen and red, and there may be small amounts of blood on the diaper. There may also be a slight yellow discharge or crust after a couple of days. Although this is normal after the procedure, some other issues are not. It is recommended that parents who choose circumcision call the doctor right away if noticing any of the following:
- Persistent bleeding or blood on diaper (more than quarter-sized)
- Persistent redness more than five days after circumcision
- Yellow discharge lasting more than a week
- Foul-smelling drainage

- Trouble urinating
- Abnormal urination within 12 hours after the circumcision
- Increasing redness, fever, or other signs of infection, such as worsening swelling or discharge, or presence of pus-filled blisters

Just like boys have the glans over the penis, girls have the labia over the vagina.

COMPLICATIONS FROM THE SURGERY:
(doctorsopposingcircumcision.com)

"The hundreds of boys I have seen who needed surgery to repair problems caused by their circumcisions are real. The men who lost more parts of their penis than the foreskin are real. The thousands of adult men saying they wish they hadn't been cut are real. Not recognizing that circumcision is harmful is either ignorance or denial." – Adrienne Carmack, M.D., urologist

There is no nationwide, standardized, prospective system in the United States or Canada for collecting data on circumcision complications in children, not even for the most severe outcomes. Therefore, no one knows how many babies require re-hospitalization, intravenous antibiotics, or a blood transfusion; how many lose all or part of their penis (beyond the foreskin); how many need repeat surgery, or how many die as a result of being circumcised. This has ethical and practical implications. Without such information, healthcare professionals are unable to inform parents of the procedure's risks adequately, and parents are subsequently unable to give truly informed consent. Physicians learning the procedure often receive little or no formal training, nor is there any legal requirement for such.

Bleeding, infection and the removal of either too much or too little skin are the most common complications for circumcisions. Further complications include: hemorrhage, scarring, difficulty urinating, damage to the urethra, partial or complete loss of the glans or penis, urinary retention, dislocation of the Plastibell ring, hematoma, multiple pyogenic granulomas, subglanular stricture, scrotal trauma, leg cyanosis, gastric rupture, pulmonary embolism, pneumothorax, erythema multiforme, myocardial injury, tachycardia, heart failure, meatitis and meatal stenosis, adhesions and skin bridges, phimosis, buried or trapped penis, need for repeat surgery, chordee, penile torsion, keloid formation, epidermal inclusion cysts, lymphedema, cancer in the circumcision scar, and subcutaneous granuloma, death.

〜

Note: The primary obstacle to obtaining an accurate estimate of the incidence of death from circumcision is the underreporting of circumcision as a cause or contributor to death. Instead of listing circumcision as a cause of death, the sepsis or hemorrhage/exsanguination that led to the baby's demise may instead be listed. Incomplete and inaccurate death certificates for pediatric deaths are not uncommon.

PSYCHOLOGICAL EFFECTS

"The circumcision of children has myriad negative psychological consequences that the CDC has failed to consider. Removing healthy tissue in the absence of any medical need harms the patient and is a breach of medical providers' ethical duty to the child. We believe that all people have a right to bodily autonomy and self-determination and deeply respect this fundamental tenet of international human rights law. As children cannot advocate for themselves, they need adults to understand the complexities of their emotional experiences and provide them special protection." – Psychology Today

Evidence indicates that the ability to learn and remember is present from before birth, and newborn infants have fully functioning pain pathways. The following are things to consider:

1. Circumcision causes immediate harm and trauma
2. Pain from circumcision in infancy alters the brain
3. Infant circumcision has long-term consequences for men
4. By encouraging circumcision, medical professionals are shaming boys' bodies
5. Forced genital cutting is a direct experience of sexual violence

Based on feedback from circumcised men, other potential long-term psychological effects of circumcision include reduced emotional expression, excessive or inappropriate anger, shame, shyness, fear, powerlessness, distrust, low self-esteem, increased difficulty identifying and expressing feelings and decreased ability for emotional intimacy. Because circumcision is generally performed shortly after birth, it is a perinatal trauma, and several authors report that perinatal trauma may contribute to self-destructive behavior in adult life. A large Danish study found that circumcised boys may have a greater risk of developing autism spectrum disorder before age ten and a higher risk for infantile autism before age five.

Changes in infant-maternal interaction have been observed after circumcision, including disrupted feeding and weaker attachment between the infant and mother. The American Academy of Pediatrics Task Force on Circumcision (1989) noted that the behavior of nearly 90 percent of circumcised infants significantly changed after the circumcision. Differences in sleep patterns and more irritability—both signs of stress—have been observed among circumcised infants.

QUESTIONS TO ASK YOURSELF IF YOU ARE CONSIDERING/PLANNING TO MUTILATE YOUR CHILD'S GENITALS:

1. Would you perform the procedure yourself?
2. Do you feel it is the child's decision as to whether they can keep what was given to them by the universe? *i.e.,* their body, their choice
3. Are you aware that the area of tissue removed from their penis will become the equivalent in size of 15 U.S. quarters when he becomes an adult?
4. Do you support female genital mutilation? Would you remove the labia if you were having a girl?
5. Are you aware of the risks involved, both immediate and long-term effects?
6. Do you understand the psychological damage it will do to their person?
7. Is inflicting pain on your newborn really how you want to begin your role as parent/protector?

8. Do you realize you are paying someone to injure your baby?
9. Do you feel comfortable consenting for another person for the removal of a body part?

"It builds confidence and strength in the mother, knowing she is there to protect him like a mother wolf would bite you if you were going to cut her baby cub." – Tiffany Leigh Crim, doula, midwife assistant

WHO IS "INTACT AMERICA?"

Intact America is the largest national advocacy group working to end involuntary circumcision in America and to ensure a healthy sexual future for all people. They fulfill their mission by challenging social and sexual norms and by advocating for the health and wellbeing of all children and the adults they will become. Intact America envisions a world where children are free from medically unnecessary surgeries carried out on them without their consent in the name of culture, religion, profit, or parental preference.

TOP 10 REASONS TO *NOT* CIRCUMCISE A BABY BOY

1. **There is no medical reason for "routine" circumcision of baby boys.** No professional medical association in the US or the rest of the world recommends routine neonatal circumcision. The American Medical Association calls it "non-therapeutic." At no time in its 75 years has the American Academy of Pediatrics ever recommended infant circumcision.
2. **The foreskin is not a birth defect.** It is a normal, sensitive, functional part of the body. In infant boys, the foreskin is attached to the head of the penis, protecting it from urine, feces, and irritation, and keeps contaminants from entering the urinary tract. The foreskin also has an important role in sexual pleasure, due to its specialized, erogenous nerve endings and its natural gliding and lubricating functions.
3. **You wouldn't circumcise your baby girl.** In the United States girls of all ages are protected from forced genital surgery by federal and state laws whether practiced in medical or non-medical settings, and

regardless of the religious or cultural preferences of their parents. There is no ethical rationale for distinguishing between female and male genital alteration. If it is unethical to remove part of a baby girl's healthy genitals, so too is it to do the same to those of a baby boy.

4. **Your baby does not want to be circumcised.** Circumcision painfully and permanently alters a baby boy's genitals, removing healthy, protective, functional tissue from the penis and exposing the child to unnecessary pain and medical risks—for no medical benefit.

5. **Removing part of a baby's penis is painful, risky, and harmful.** We know babies are sensitive to pain. Many circumcisions are performed with no analgesic, but even when pain control is employed, the pain is not eliminated. As with any surgery, complications can and do occur with circumcision (see above). All circumcisions result in the loss of the foreskin and its functions, and leave a penile scar.

6. **Times and attitudes have changed.** The circumcision rate in the United States is now somewhere around 55% (and much lower in some parts of the country), down from 81% in 1981. This means that nearly half of all baby boys leave the hospital intact, as more and more parents are realizing that circumcision is unnecessary and harmful.

7. **Most medically advanced nations do not circumcise baby boys.** People in Europe, Asia and Latin America are often appalled to hear that American doctors and hospitals remove part of a boy's penis shortly after birth. Approximately 75% of the men in the world are not circumcised and remain intact throughout their lives.

8. **Caring for and cleaning the foreskin is easy.** A natural, intact penis requires no special care beyond gentle washing while bathing. Later, when the foreskin can be retracted, a boy can be taught to move back his foreskin to wash his penis. Forcible retraction of the foreskin results in pain and injury.

9. **Circumcision does not prevent HIV or other diseases.** Over the years, the claims that circumcision prevents various diseases have repeatedly been proven to be exaggerated or outright fabrications. Most men in the United States are circumcised, but our STD rates are as high as or higher than those in countries where circumcision is rare.

10. **Children should be protected from permanent bodily alteration inflicted on them without their consent in the name of culture, religion, profit, or parental preference.** Under accepted bioethical principles, parents can consent to surgery on behalf of a child only if it is necessary to protect the child's life or health. "Routine" circumcision fails this test because it painfully and permanently removes a normal and healthy part of a boy's penis, does not protect the child's life or health, and in fact creates new risks. Removing the foreskin is no more justified than removing a finger or any other healthy body part.

THE MYTHS & FACTS BEHIND CIRCUMCISION

Myth – Circumcising baby boys is a safe and harmless procedure.

Fact – Surgically removing part of a baby boy's penis causes pain, creates immediate health risks and can lead to serious complications, which can and do occur in even the best clinical settings.

Myth – Circumcision is just a little snip.

Fact – Surgical removal of the foreskin involves immobilizing the baby by strapping him face-up onto a molded plastic board. In one common method, the doctor then inserts a metal instrument under the foreskin to forcibly separate it from the glans, slits the foreskin, and inserts a circumcision device. The foreskin is crushed and then cut off. The amount of skin removed in a typical infant circumcision is the equivalent of 15 square inches in an adult male.

Myth – The baby does not feel any pain during circumcision.

Fact – Circumcision is painful. Babies are sensitive to pain, just like older children and adults. The analgesics used for circumcision only decrease pain; they do not eliminate it. If the baby is not crying while it is happening, the baby is likely experiencing shock, and is disassociating from what is happening in order to survive. The open wound left by the removal of the foreskin will continue to cause the baby pain and discomfort for the 7–10 days it takes to heal.

Myth – If I don't circumcise my son, he will be ridiculed.

Fact – Times have changed and so has people's understanding of circumcision. Most medically advanced nations do not practice child circumcision. Three quarters of the world's men are intact.

Myth – A boy should be circumcised to look like his father.

Fact – Children differ from their parents in many ways, including eye and hair color, body type, and (of course) size and sexual development. If a child asks why his penis looks different from that of his circumcised father (or brother), parents can say, "Daddy (or brother) had a part of his penis removed when he was a baby; now we know it's not necessary, and we decided to not hire someone to do that to you."

Myth – Routine circumcision of baby boys cannot be compared to Female Genital Mutilation.

Fact – Rationales offered in cultures that promote female genital cutting — hygiene, disease prevention, improved appearance of the genitalia, and social acceptance—are similar to those offered in cultures that promote male circumcision. Whatever the rationale, forced removal of healthy genital tissue from any child—male or female—is unethical. Boys have the same right as girls to an intact body, and to be spared this inhumane, unnecessary surgery.

Myth – To oppose male circumcision is religious and cultural bigotry.

Fact – Many who oppose the permanent alteration of children's genitals do so because they believe in universal human rights. All children—regardless of their ethnicity or culture—have the right to be protected from bodily harm.

Myth – Circumcising newborn baby boys produces health benefits later in life.

Fact – There is NO link between circumcision and better health. In fact, cutting a baby boy's genitals creates immediate health risks. The foreskin is actually an important and functional body part, protecting the head of the penis from injury and providing moisture and lubrication. Circumcision also diminishes sexual pleasure later in life.

Myth – Male circumcision helps prevent HIV.

Fact – Claims that circumcision prevents HIV have repeatedly been proven to be exaggerated or false. Only abstinence or safe sex, including the use of condoms, can prevent the spread of sexually transmitted diseases, including HIV/AIDS.

"... I asked a friend if he felt 'different' when he was the only uncircumcised man in the shower and he said, 'Yes, gloriously different." – Kristen O'Hara

FORESKIN RESTORATION

"...I'm restoring my foreskin because I was born with one, and damn it, I'm going to die with one." – Jim Bigelow, PHD, *The Joy of Uncircumsizing*

Foreskin restoration is the process of expanding the skin on the penis to reconstruct an organ similar to the foreskin, which has been removed by circumcision. Restoration creates a facsimile of the foreskin, but specialized tissues removed during circumcision cannot be reclaimed. Actual regeneration of the foreskin is experimental at this time. Surgical methods, known as foreskin reconstruction, usually involve a method of grafting skin (taken from the scrotum) onto the distal portion of the penile shaft. Such techniques are costly, and have the potential to produce unsatisfactory results or serious complications related to the skin graft.

British Columbia resident Paul Tinari was held down and circumcised at the age of eight in what he stated was "a routine form of punishment" for masturbation at residential schools. Following a lawsuit, the British Columbia Ministry of Health paid for Tinari's surgical foreskin restoration. The plastic surgeon who performed the restoration was the first in Canada to have done such an operation, and used a technique similar to the above described.

JUDAISM
Many people will state religion as a reason they are mutilating the child. When I asked a Jewish mother why she did it, she responded that it was in the bible. So I looked for a passage and found the following.

The commandment to circumcise is given in Genesis 17:10-14: "For the generations to come every male among you who is eight days old must be circumcised, including those born in your household or bought with money from a foreigner—those who are not your offspring. Whether born in your household or bought with your money, they must be circumcised."

Leviticus 12:3 also states: "And in the eighth day the flesh of his foreskin shall be circumcised."

Interestingly enough, the bible also contains the first sign of evidence for uncircumcision among the Jews. It can be seen in a passage of the Old Testament (I Maccabees 1: 14-15): "Whereupon they built a place of exercise at Jerusalem according to the customs of the heathen. And made themselves uncircumcised (sibi praeputia fecerunt), and forsook the holy covenant, and joined themselves to the heathen, and were sold to do mischief." This passage was written at the time of the reign of Antiochus IV (168 BC), when the hellenization of Palestine and, therefore, the oppression of the Jewish religion and culture came to a first climax. Hellenistic ideals gained popularity, and it was, for example, common to exhibit the naked body at athletic games or at public baths. Jews were forced to hide their genitalia or restore their foreskins, so as not to be persecuted and to improve their social and economic position. This situation culminated in a law by Antiochius dictating that the act of circumcision was to be punished by death sentence.

> (I Maccabees 1:63-64): "Now the women that circumcised their children, were slain according to the commandment of king Antiochus. And they hanged the children about their necks in all their houses: and those that had circumcised them, they put to death."

So, the passages also contain the buying of babies, slaying of mothers, hanging of children, and death for those who had done the circumcising. I wonder why these parts of the passages aren't mentioned as often?

A BRIS

A bris is the Jewish ceremony where the baby boy, at 8 days old, is circumcised by a mohel, a rabbi who specializes in performing circumcisions. The Bible does not specify a reason for the choice of the eighth day; however, modern medicine has revealed that an infant's blood clotting mechanism stabilizes on the eighth day after birth. As with almost any commandment, circumcision can be postponed for health reasons. Jewish law provides that when the child's health is at issue, circumcision must wait until 7 days after a doctor declares the child healthy enough to undergo the procedure.

While the circumcision is performed, the child is held by the "sandek." In English, this is often referred to as godfather. The sandek is usually a grandparent or family rabbi.

INTERVIEW WITH A MAN WHO HELD HIS NEPHEW AT A BRIS

What was the experience like for you on that day when you held your nephew as he was circumcised?

"Ultimately it turned out to be a very horrifying experience. There were mostly men except for my sister, my nephew's mother. There was a very stern environment, very matter of fact, very dark. It didn't feel celebratory."

Can you describe the baby's experience of the event?

"Well, as you can imagine, he did not want to have anything to do with it. What was particularly horrifying was that it was my job to hold the child. So they handed me his naked body, and he was screaming and crying. My sister's face was white, and I was just thinking, 'Why is this happening?' What was extremely striking and made an imprint on my mind was that he resisted the circumcision with every fiber of his being. It was shocking how strong this eight-day-little boy was, and I had to work very hard to hold him still. I remember breaking a sweat. And I remember at that junction making a decision that if I ever had a baby boy, I would never put him through that ordeal or willfully ask someone else to do it."

I think in the hospital they tie them down to some sort of board. You have had a son recently and I am wondering, because your family is Jewish, did your family object to your not having your son circumcised?

"No, not really. They had come to expect unconventional things from me, so it wasn't a surprise, nor did they make an argument. I told them that after the experience that I had had with my nephew that it was barbaric and there was no way. There was no reason to do it. It damages the child, and it is just horrifying. It is insane to think that we put people through this and willfully create suffering in this life."

What did your pediatrician think?
"To my surprise, she was elated. I wouldn't have been surprised if she had started jumping up and down for joy, she was so happy that we had made the decision not to circumcise him."

> "I have not performed a circumcision since 1994. It is a cruel, unnecessary and…substandard practice which belongs in the history books, not in the hospital or the clinic." – Steven Dorfman, MD, pediatrician

CUTTING BABIES IN THE NAME OF RELIGIOUS TRADITION

There has been an enormous amount of pain caused in the name of religion. Wars have been fought, people killed, boys raped by priests, women treated horribly, etc.

There has been a lot of pain caused in the name of "tradition." Tradition, by definition, is the transmission of customs or beliefs from generation to generation, or the fact of being passed on in this way; a doctrine believed to have authority. Doing something because it is tradition doesn't make something okay. Doing something because ancestors did it doesn't make something okay. Tradition doesn't mean that it is moral or ethical. It's an American tradition to eat turkeys on thanksgiving. Slaughtering millions of innocent creatures on a day of expressing gratitude for life doesn't mean it is compassionate. It is tradition in some gangs to kill a person for membership. It is tradition for fraternities to "haze" their pledges with their rituals of harassment, humiliation, and abuse, which, in some cases, lead to death.

FEMALE CIRCUMCISION / FEMALE GENITAL MUTILATION

We hear a lot about male circumcision, but rarely do we hear about female circumcision, most often called female genital mutilation, or FGM. FGM refers to all procedures involving partial or total removal of the external female genitalia or other injury to the female genital organs for cultural or other non-medical reasons. Female genital mutilation is a criminal offense in 27 states in the US. If you visit the US Department of State website, you will find the following statement: "The U.S. Government considers FGM/C to be a serious human rights abuse, and a form of gender-based violence and child abuse." Why wouldn't the cutting of males be "gender-based violence" as well? If you search their site for a statement concerning MGM, you will not find one.

ORIGINS OF FGM

The origins of the practice are unclear. It predates the rise of Christianity and Islam. It is said that some Egyptian mummies display characteristics of FGM. Historians claim that, in the fifth century BC, the Phoenicians, the Hittites and the Ethiopians practiced circumcision. It is also reported that circumcision rites were practiced in Africa, the Philippines, by certain tribes in the Upper Amazon, Australia, and by early Romans and Arabs. As recent as the 1950s, clitoridectomy has been practiced in Western Europe and the United States.

AGE IT IS PERFORMED

In some areas, FGM is carried out during infancy—as early as a couple of days after birth. In others, it takes place during childhood, at the time of marriage, during a woman's first pregnancy or after the birth of her first child. Recent reports suggest that the age has been dropping in some areas, with most FGM carried out on girls between the ages of 0 and 15 years.

SERIOUS IMPLICATIONS FOR GIRLS AND WOMEN INCLUDE:

- severe pain
- shock
- hemorrhage
- tetanus
- infections
- ulceration of the genitals and injury to adjacent tissue
- fever
- septicemia
- anemia
- formation of cysts and abscesses
- damage to the urethra
- sexual dysfunction
- increased risk of HIV transmission
- complications during childbirth
- severe scar formation
- difficulty in urinating
- menstrual disorders
- infertility
- and of course psychological effects.

Infibulation is the practice of excising the clitoris and labia of a girl or woman and stitching together the edges of the vulva to prevent sexual intercourse, which creates a physical barrier to sexual intercourse and childbirth. An infibulated woman therefore has to undergo gradual dilation of the vaginal opening before sexual intercourse can take place. Often, infibulated women are cut open on the first night of marriage (by the husband or a circumciser), to enable the husband to be intimate with his wife. At childbirth, many women also have to be cut again because the vaginal opening is too small to allow for the passage of a baby. If this is making you feel sick, sad, angry, or all of the above, it is a good sign of your compassion.

WHY IS SO MUCH CUTTING GOING ON?

Male and female genital mutilation, episiotomies, C-sections, wrists, teens cutting for psychological reasons, and ultimately, we are cutting ourselves off from our true self, our wisdom, love, empathy and compassion.

Q&A ON THE STREETS

While recording my radio show, I took to local sidewalks and parks to approach various people, men and women, to ask their thoughts on circumcision. They did not know me, and I simply asked if they would answer a question or two. The following "interviews" are transcribed below.

LADY IN PARK

What are your thoughts on male circumcision? I think it's normal. In the US all males are [circumcised], so it's normal.

The skin there was placed by mistake? I don't know.

Why do you think it's there if it's just going to be cut off? I don't think there's a purpose for it. I've never seen an uncircumcised penis.

How do you feel about FGM? I think that's wrong. I don't think they should be cutting them.

What's the difference between the two? I don't think we cut females vaginas like they do in Africa. I think it's for male power. Controlling.

If you had a boy would you have him circumcised? Yeah.

Would you be able to do it yourself? No.

How come? I don't want to hurt him.

GUY IN PARK

What are your thoughts on male circumcision? I think it is -wow- it's very illegal and disgusting. It's unthinkable and inexcusable. God, no.

So I imagine your feelings on FGM are similar? Yeah. Pretty gruesome stuff.

Can you tell me why you wouldn't? Because I haven't been [circumcised], so I don't want to do it to my son if I have one. For me, I wouldn't do it.

Did you ever wonder why you weren't, or why other boys were? Was it an issue when you were growing up? No.

GUY IN BLACK T-SHIRT

Can you tell me how you feel about male circumcision? I got it done. Normal thing to do.

And if you had a child? I guess. It's normal here.

If it weren't normal, would you not do it? I don't know, honestly. I never had to think about it.

So, if it were done to you later in life, age 10, you would have chosen to have it done? I don't know. I'm big against going to the doctor. It's a fight to make me go for medicine. They made me go for shots, and I thought that was normal also. Maybe.

Do you think that cutting the skin off the penis would be painful? There would be ways to get around the pain and the recuperating after. Same with any operation.

Any other thoughts? I never thought about it.

JEWISH MOTHER

Did you circumcise your son? I did.

Why? Cause it's the covenant with Abraham and God, and we follow Jewish religion.

Why? Health reasons. Children are tough. I don't want him to be worried about cleaning under his foreskin.

Do you know where that instruction comes from? Other than the Bible, I don't. Abraham was one of our great masters, and he had a contract, and we fulfill it because we are Jewish.

How do you feel about Female Genital Mutilation? It's horrible. They do it when they are 12 or 13, so there is a lot of pain.

What if the male had to be that age when circumcised? My husband was and it was very painful. I don't think he would have chosen to do it. He didn't have a choice though. He was 13.

TALL SKINNY GUY

What are your thoughts on male circumcision? I think it's a strange practice to have to continue in this day and age. Doesn't make a lot of sense any more. A cultural practice. If god made me this way, why should we take that away?

Do you have children? No.

If you had a son would you? I would not.

Do you know why people do it? I think I know why. It's to keep it easier to clean. Maybe back in the day, but apparently that is the reason people give.

How do you feel about FGM? I know that it's still practiced today. I don't hear about it that much, but people are usually outraged about it. I don't know why that's practiced, but it seems like a not very compassionate thing to do, either.

GUY #2 IN PARK

Do you mind telling me your thoughts on circumcision? Okay.

If you had the choice to do it as opposed to your mother and father choosing? Yeah, I would have.

Best to do as a newborn or later in life? At birth, because I've heard it's harder getting it done as an adult.

More painful? Would you think that would be the case? I am [circumcised], and both my sons were at birth.

Could you have done it to your sons? Myself? No.

What about FGM? I don't agree with that.

Can you tell me why? I don't think it's right. I don't know much about it. Why would they do that to begin with?

JENNIFER

What do you know about male circumcision? I know my husband isn't and is very grateful. It's a seemingly ancient practice, because most of the nerve endings are on that piece. We have talked about it. He was born in England. People use the argument of cleanliness. It's not that hard to keep an intact penis clean.

If you had a child would you? No, I don't believe so. It's similar to the female circumcision that goes on.

ALICE

Did you have your son circumcised? I did.

What was the reason? I'm embarrassed that I didn't take the time to research it. My mother is a nurse, my brother a pediatrician...not getting made fun of in the locker room.

What do you think of female circumcision? That sounds terrible.

THOMAS

Do you mind telling me your thoughts on circumcision? I am a proud owner of a circumcised penis.

If you had the choice, would you have chosen to do that? In retrospect, I just like what I have.

How do you feel about it in general? I guess since you're so young, it's a choice made for you. That's what's weird about it. Everyone seems to like what they got.

Do you know why it's done? I don't know why. Probably used to be health reasons.

CHERYL

Do you have any boys? Yes.

Are they circumcised? It was a long time ago, and their father was rather insistent, and it was a hard decision on my part, but I decided to do it, so they could fit in with extended family and cousins.

WOMAN IN BLACK SHIRT

Do you mind telling me your thoughts on circumcision? It doesn't make a difference to me.

If you had a son? Probably.

Would you do it yourself? No. I wouldn't be able to inflict pain on my own child. I would rather someone else do it and [I] not be in there.

And why would you have it done? Um, basically because they tell you it's more normal.

So, why do you think that the foreskin is there if it's supposed to come off? No idea.

How do you feel about FGM? I don't even know what it is. I've never heard of it before.

GUY #3 IN PARK

Do you mind telling me your thoughts on circumcision? I believe it's healthy, the flap over the penis. When you have sex, stuff could get in there.

Uncircumcised is healthy? Yeah, I think so.

How do you feel about FGM? I did not know that females had it.

MALE CIRCUMCISION DECREASES PENILE SENSITIVITY & SEXUAL PLEASURE

Experts (and guys) claim that circumcision can reduce sexual sensation, as the procedure removes thousands of nerve endings in the penis. In fact, a 2007 study found that the glans of the uncircumcised penis was more sensitive to light touch than the glans of a circumcised penis. In addition to increased sensation to the glans, the extra skin adds more friction and stimulation to the clitoris during penetration (both get extra pleasure).

OBJECTIVE: To test the hypothesis that sensitivity of the foreskin is a substantial part of male penile sensitivity.

STUDY: The study consisted of 1359 men via an online survey. Respondents were recruited by means of leaflets and advertising.

RESULTS: The analysis sample consisted of 1059 uncircumcised and 310 circumcised men. For the glans penis, circumcised men reported decreased sexual pleasure and lower orgasm intensity. They also stated more effort was required to achieve orgasm, and a higher percentage of them experienced unusual sensations (burning, prickling, itching, or tingling and numbness of the glans penis). For the penile shaft a higher percentage of circumcised men described discomfort and pain, numbness and unusual sensations. In comparison to men circumcised before puberty, men circumcised during adolescence or later indicated less sexual pleasure at the glans penis, and a higher percentage of them reported discomfort or pain and unusual sensations at the penile shaft.

CONCLUSION: This study confirms the importance of the foreskin for penile sensitivity, overall sexual satisfaction, and penile functioning. Furthermore, this study shows that a higher percentage of circumcised men experience discomfort or pain and unusual sensations as compared with the uncircumcised population.

Study by: Department of Urology, Ghent University Hospital, Ghent, Belgium, May 2013

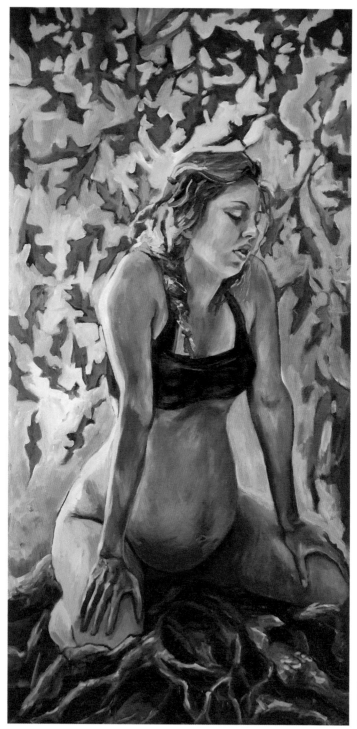

224

CHAPTER 15:
VBAC (VAGINAL BIRTH AFTER CESAREAN)

"My OB put it in perspective for me. He's seen 1 uterine rupture in 29 years...and she had not previously had a C-section."
- VANESSA SPAHAN
A Birth Without Fear Mama

"Your body is not a lemon!" Believe in your body's ability to birth. You may have received messages from your prior birth that made you doubt birth or feel like you failed somehow. You did not fail. Do whatever work it takes prenatally to help you rediscover – or discover for the first time – the power and strength you have within you to birth."
- INA MAY GASKIN

"I was in such shock and filled with more joy and gratitude and healing than ever before in my life. I couldn't believe I did it, even though I knew I could. I achieved my VBAC. I had worked my butt off mentally, physically and spiritually. I am forever thankful for my support systems."
- RANDI SHEPPARD,
Mother

A WOMAN WHO DESIRES to birth their child vaginally, but has had a previous Cesarean operation, may find it difficult to locate a supportive doctor or hospital. State laws can prohibit some midwives from attending VBACs. Only four states do not allow VBACs at home with licensed midwives. They are Alaska, Arizona, Arkansas, and my home state, South Carolina. Women are pressured so often into having a repeat Cesarean, that when calling the ICAN organization, there is the option to "Press three if you feel you're being forced into a C-section." If pressed, it will then ask the caller to "press two if currently in labor." From there, she is connected to a volunteer representative with a medical or legal background.

In 1980, a consensus of experts called by the National Institutes of Health said vaginal births after prior Caesareans should be an option for women. In 1988, the American College of Obstetricians and Gynecologists went further, saying that unless there were medical reasons for surgery, pregnant women with previous Caesareans should be encouraged to deliver vaginally.

Data from large clinical studies have demonstrated the safety and success of VBAC with proper care. So why then are so many women told by their doctor that if they had a Cesarean with their first, all subsequent births must be C-sections?

IMPORTANT TO KNOW ABOUT VBAC

THE LABOR IS NORMAL

Do everything to prepare for a normal labor. Two keys are to choose your support and place of birth carefully. The culture of the hospital and the clinical judgment calls made by your doctor or midwife can make all the difference, so make sure you feel comfortable with them. What is your gut telling you after your appointments? Trust your intuition. Change providers if it doesn't feel right. The sooner, the better, but even late in the pregnancy, you can always change your mind/heart. Educate yourself, know your options, hire a doula if you can, and learn relaxation tools. Labor in the comfort of your home until you're in active labor (4–7cm), and if you're able to avoid interventions, you increase your chances for a successful VBAC.

UTERINE RUPTURE IS THE MAJOR FEAR ASSOCIATED

One of the biggest fears and main deterrents in the VBAC decision is uterine rupture. Uterine rupture is when the uterus tears. It can tear along a prior cesarean scar, OR it can happen in an un-scarred (read: no previous cesarean) uterus. The studies put the incidence of uterine rupture at .07% of all births (which includes moms with no scar on their uterus and VBAC moms). Only looking at VBAC moms, the rate is higher at a still-low .3%–.7%, depending upon the study. A 2009 systemic review with meta-analysis of success rate and adverse outcomes of VBAC after two cesareans (VBAC2) vs. VBAC after one cesarean showed a uterine rupture rate in VBAC2 of 1.36% (and a success rate of 71.1% for VBAC2).

I have seen one uterine rupture as a doula. The mother was started on Pitocin, which increases the risks of rupture. Her uterus had been contracting consistently for many hours without much of a break in between. Her body was working for her and no longer needed augmentation with drugs; therefore, the nurses were asked to turn down or turn off the Pitocin, and it was turned down. She was at 8 cm dilation when things shifted.

The fetal monitors strapped around the belly tend to move around, and the nurse at one point came in to fix them so that they could get a proper reading on the fetal heartbeat. The nurse aggressively undid the Velcro on the belts to remove them, and in the process, hit the mother's belly (and she yelped in pain). Then the nurse did it again! She was not taking enough care to be gentle. Immediately after that, the mother began complaining of a sharp abdominal pain that persisted. Her mother's intuition was telling her something was wrong. Shortly after that, the doctor placed an electrode directly on the fetal scalp through the cervix (an internal fetal monitor) to evaluate the fetal heart rate and variability between beats. Because the mother sensed the baby was in danger, she cried out to have them perform a C-section so that her baby would be okay. She was immediately taken to the operating room. She was right. Her uterus had ruptured.

The father was not allowed to go with her down the hall and into the OR with her. He was left with us in the room, crying, waiting to be called into the operation, and feeling helpless while his wife was now alone and in pain.

I believe the Pitocin and hard hits to the belly were two of the causes for the uterine rupture. After the operation, the mother and baby were both okay. The baby was strong, alert, and beautiful. The mother was courageous, relieved, and beautiful.

Studies/Statistics: birthwithoutfear.com
Publication on Uterine Rupture: Medscape.com
Uterine rupture rates: VBAC.com

IF THE DOCTOR SCHEDULES A CESAREAN, THAT IS NOT SUPPORTIVE OF A VBAC

Many women will exclaim how they love their doctor who is so supportive of their VBAC—"He told me I could do whatever I want,"—just before they state the date of their scheduled Cesarean. The doctor is NOT supportive if he or she has planned a C-section "just in case" at a certain (arbitrary) week of gestation, often before 40 weeks. If a good candidate for a VBAC (most women are), then it is a normal labor and should be treated as such. If you happen to be in the 10–20% of moms whose TOLAC (trial of labor after Cesarean) results in a repeat cesarean, they will find an operating room. If in the prior labor(s) the mother's cervix dilated, the body holds that memory, which will help in a VBAC labor. If not, the labor is considered like a first birth. The process unfolds best if the mother allows the body to go into labor spontaneously. The mother should talk beforehand with her provider about options and desires in the case of a necessary repeat cesarean.

STUDIES SUPPORT THEM

Studies show that 75–90% of women who attempt a VBAC successfully have a vaginal birth; for numerous reasons, only about 8% of women try. Is it because of the fear of uterine rupture? Or because she isn't fully informed about VBAC benefits and risks as well as the contrasting benefits and risks of repeat cesarean? Lack of knowledge produces tension and fear, which is never conducive to good decision-making.

12 OF THE QUESTIONS ASKED ABOUT VBAC:

The care provider, to ensure she is a good candidate for VBAC, may ask a pregnant mother who is seeking a vaginal delivery after Cesarean:

1. When is your baby due?
2. Can you provide a copy of your operative report? (to find out if the uterus was closed with a double layer of sutures)
3. Reason your baby was delivered by cesarean? Fetal stress? Failure to progress? Other? Please describe the details.
4. How many weeks along into your pregnancy were you?
5. How dilated were you before they decided to do the cesarean?

6. Did you heal without any infection after the cesarean?
7. How much did your baby weigh?
8. How old is your baby now?
9. Are you in good health and having a normal pregnancy this time?
10. What is your height and weight?
11. Have you had any vaginal births?
12. How many cesareans have you had?

WHY DON'T DOCTORS SUPPORT THEM?

Some physicians are not comfortable with a mother attempting a vaginal birth after one C-section. Many physicians will not agree to be the attending if a mother has had two C-sections. Not many physicians at all will attend a VBAC if a mother has had three or four C-sections. But, it is essential to remember that it is ultimately the choice of the mother.

Other factors that prevent support:

- A vertical incision from previous C-section, which shows a higher risk of uterine rupture. (a transverse incision has lower risk)
- Health complications, such as a heart defect or lung disease, because an emergency C-section can be dangerous with these conditions
- Having a large baby (important to note that estimated fetus size is not exact and many moms vaginally birth babies over 10 pounds)
- Going past the due date
- Threat of lawsuits

ARE THEY LEGAL?

VBAC's are NOT illegal anywhere in the USA.

It is legal to have a hospital VBAC in all 50 states.

It is legal to have an out-of-hospital VBAC in all 50 states.

If someone has told you that VBAC is illegal, they are either misinformed or are outright lying to you. Ask them to show you the law stating that it is illegal. This is something you should be able to look up through a quick Internet search. But you won't find it because it doesn't exist.

What may not be "allowed" by state regulation or law varies from state to state, but if restrictions are present, it is in the form of restrictions on the license or practice of the practitioner if she is a midwife; MDs can do what they want. But if the hospital that the doctor practices it won't offer it, then they are restricted.

Birth Centers with a license from their state often have restrictions specified in the law or their regulations (force of law), which mean they could lose their license in regards to certain situations (such as VBAC, breech, multiples). Their state regulatory board decides these situations and restrictions.

Some states, like New Jersey, permit midwives to attend homebirths, but not homebirth VBACs (HBACs). In other states, like California, homebirth and HBAC are legal for midwives to attend, though you technically need to use your right of informed refusal to have an HBAC. Some states have laws prohibiting midwifery care, like North Carolina, and in those states, a Home Birth After Cesarean would be considered illegal for them to attend.

HOSPITAL POLICIES OF VBAC
Once again, it is legal to have a hospital VBAC in all 50 states. But some hospitals simply do not support them. Full Circle Midwifery's website contains a state-by-state VBAC policy summary, researched in 2009, where information was collected to identify VBAC policies in individual hospitals, to reveal the hospitals that have official bans against VBAC in place. Other hospitals have de facto bans in place, which means the hospital indicates there is no official policy against VBAC, but in reality, there are no doctors there who will agree to attend one, or the restrictions on a VBAC are so extreme that it is highly unlikely a VBAC would be achieved. The research concluded that no more than 10% of the hospitals they spoke to are indeed VBAC supportive. In regards to individual OBGYN views on VBACs, that would be more difficult to attain, but what I hear most from mothers is, "I have to have a second C-section because I already had one."

VBAC CONSENT FORM
Many hospitals will ask the mother to sign a consent form stating that she understands the benefits and risks of both a VBAC and a Cesarean operation. Read through the form carefully. One mother I was a doula for, was reading through the form, at 36 weeks pregnant, and realized it said "I

am required to receive an epidural during the active phase of labor." She asked the provider, who said yes, that is "non-negotiable." The mother did not sign the form, and contacted me to express her apprehension. I had not heard of this before, and called around to other local hospitals to find out what their form said. It surprised me that a facility would state that it was mandatory for a mother to inject drugs into her body. No other local hospital required the epidural. The mother called another hospital for an appointment, and several days later, met with a new care provider who was supportive of her decision to try and birth naturally.

SAMPLE VBAC CONSENT FORM CONTENTS:

TRIAL OF LABOR AFTER CESAREAN DELIVERY (TOLAC) CONSENT FORM

You must initial each statement to show you understand.

_____I have had one or more cesarean section deliveries.

_____I am choosing to have labor and deliver by vaginal birth, rather than choosing a repeat cesarean section birth.

_____This hospital does not offer the highest level of services for vaginal deliveries for women who have had cesarean section deliveries with other pregnancies.

_____About 60–80% of women who try to deliver vaginally after a cesarean section will deliver vaginally.

_____The benefits of a vaginal birth with no complications include: less blood loss, less post-delivery complications, shorter recovery/healing time.

_____The risk of a rupture of the uterus during labor is about 1% (or 1 in 100) vaginal deliveries. This is with an incision in my uterus from the cesarean section before. Labor poses a higher risk of harm to my baby than to me. If there is a rupture in my uterus, my baby may suffer brain damage or death, if not immediately delivered by emergency cesarean section.

_____If my uterus ruptures during labor, I understand there may not be enough time to operate and prevent death or permanent brain injury to my baby.

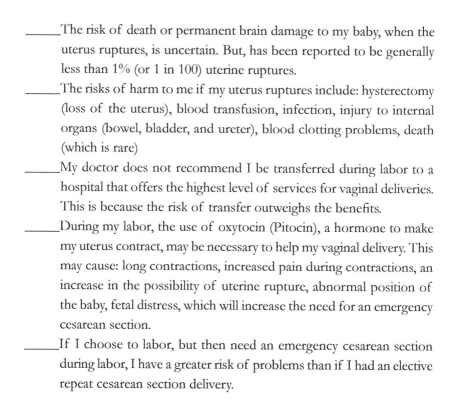

_____The risk of death or permanent brain damage to my baby, when the uterus ruptures, is uncertain. But, has been reported to be generally less than 1% (or 1 in 100) uterine ruptures.

_____The risks of harm to me if my uterus ruptures include: hysterectomy (loss of the uterus), blood transfusion, infection, injury to internal organs (bowel, bladder, and ureter), blood clotting problems, death (which is rare)

_____My doctor does not recommend I be transferred during labor to a hospital that offers the highest level of services for vaginal deliveries. This is because the risk of transfer outweighs the benefits.

_____During my labor, the use of oxytocin (Pitocin), a hormone to make my uterus contract, may be necessary to help my vaginal delivery. This may cause: long contractions, increased pain during contractions, an increase in the possibility of uterine rupture, abnormal position of the baby, fetal distress, which will increase the need for an emergency cesarean section.

_____If I choose to labor, but then need an emergency cesarean section during labor, I have a greater risk of problems than if I had an elective repeat cesarean section delivery.

By signing below, I confirm I have reviewed this information. I have talked with my doctor, and have had all my questions answered. By signing this form, I give my consent to all appropriate treatment in the event of a uterine rupture or other complications, including: hysterectomy, blood transfusion for me and/or baby, emergency cesarean, and emergency resuscitation.

PREPARATION FOR A VBAC

Find care providers who support you and will do so through the labor and birth.

Hire a doula and/or a monitrice. A monitrice is a person who does what a doula does in labor and birth, but additionally has midwifery, nursing, or medical training in maternal-child health. She may be a former labor & delivery nurse, a certified professional midwife, or a non-practicing nurse-midwife, who is trained in fetal monitoring, performing cervical exams in labor, and neonatal resuscitation. A monitrice can be with the mother at home, functioning as the doula, yet also monitoring the labor and communicating with the primary health care provider, who could be a midwife or physician. A monitrice goes with the laboring woman to the hospital when she is close to birthing, and continues her support, while the woman's midwife or physician catches the baby.

Maintain a healthy diet, active lifestyle, and good weight gain.

Allowing labor to begin on its own, and refraining from interventions will contribute to a successful VBAC.

Seek out therapeutic modalities if the first birth was traumatic or difficult. Find someone who will listen to your story, which can help to release emotions like anger, sadness, or fear. Healing practices can be effective, liberating, and comforting.

- **Yoga:** asana and meditation keep the body in good health
- **Chiropractic care:** this can be useful if the pelvis is misaligned
- **Reiki:** an ancient Japanese method of hands-on healing that targets the energy fields in the body, where there has been physical or emotional pain
- **Acupuncture:** insertion of thin needles through the skin at strategic points on the body, balancing the flow of energy or life force, known as chi; an ancient Chinese method
- **Sound Therapy:** by using rhythm and frequency, the brainwaves are entrained, and it becomes possible to down-shift our normal beta state (ordinary waking consciousness) to an alpha (relaxed), theta (meditative), or delta (sleep) state, where internal healing can occur
- **Cranial Sacral Therapy:** a gentle, non-invasive therapy that focuses on the wave-like rhythmic pulse that goes through the entire body; stemming from osteopathy, which emphasizes the role of the musculoskeletal system in health and disease
- **Massage:** can enhance your overall sense of emotional and physical well-being
- **EMDR (Eye Movement Desensitization and Reprocessing):** a psychotherapy treatment that alleviates distress associated with traumatic memories to help ease tension in the body and mind.

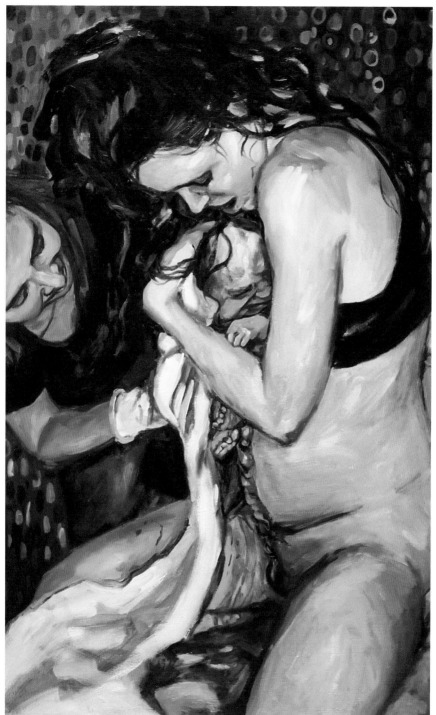

Amanda Greavette

CHAPTER 16: VERNIX

"Touch is the first language we speak."
- STEPHEN GASKIN

"Babies are not born dirty. Don't wash it off. Rub it in."
- MANY PEOPLE

"Birth is not neat and fast and quiet. It's gritty and primal."
- MAYIM BIALIK

MY SON HAS A book called "Mud," about a little boy and girl who are playing in mud and getting it all over themselves. At spas, people do mud masks, seaweed wraps, and salt scrubs. We put cleansers, oils, and creams on our faces and bodies. The cream that we are born with is better than all of this! So why wipe it off? Babies aren't born dirty. We can think of it as their first spa body treatment, free and full of goodness!

Vernix caseosa is the white, waxy, cheesy substance coating baby's skin when they appear outside of the womb. In Latin, "vernix" means to varnish, and "caseous" is a cheesy nature. Vernix begins to form on the unborn baby around 20 weeks gestation, partially to prevent baby's skin from getting too waterlogged after living in amniotic fluid for months. It is more permeable to the transport of water and other small molecules to the baby. Although it helps protect baby's skin from amniotic fluid, the creamy vernix itself contains about 80% water and many beneficial components. Scientists have identified lipids, amino acids, proteins, antibacterial, and antimicrobial compounds in vernix, including wax, sterol esters, ceramides, squalene, cholesterol, triglycerides, phospholipids, asparagine, and glutamine. About 61% of the proteins found in this white substance found only in vernix. Humans are the only ones that produce it.

BENEFITS OF VERNIX

A primary purpose of vernix is to protect the infant from unwanted pathogens, both in and out of the womb. The mucus plug and amniotic sac both help protect baby from harmful bacteria, but vernix is the last line of defense. Newborns can't control their temperature, and the vernix is a natural insulator that helps regulate it. Losing this layer of vernix too soon exposes infants to skin infections and fevers if they get too cold. The mother's body (skin to skin immediately following birth) also helps keep baby warm and regulates their temperature.

Vernix is a skin cleanser and antioxidant. It offers a protective covering as the baby goes through the birth canal. The baby picks up beneficial bacteria and potentially avoids overgrowths of harmful bacteria, viruses, and fungi in the mother's vagina, including E.coli, Staph aureus, Group B Strep, Pseudomonas aeruginosa, Candida albicana, Listeria monocytogenes, Serratia marcescens, and Klebsiella pneumonia. These pathogens can cause things like diarrhea, meningitis, and pneumonia in newborn infants.

IN THE WOMB VERNIX:
- Prevents loss of electrolytes and fluids
- Provides a protective layer to facilitate skin growth underneath
- Seals the skin to prevent the amniotic fluid from permeating it
- Acts as a microbial barrier from unwanted pathogens

OUT OF WOMB VERNIX:
- Decreases skin pH and helps form the protective acid mantle
- Protects from pathogens
- Locks moisture into skin, keeping it soft and supple
- Contains the new baby smell to help mother and baby bond when breastfeeding
- A baby's first bowel movement is a green, tar-like substance (referred to as meconium) that consists of amniotic fluid, secretions of the intestinal glands, bile pigments, fatty acids, and intrauterine debris. It can become problematic if passed before birth in some instances. The vernix plays a crucial role in helping to protect the baby from early meconium exposure.
- The mother's chest is the optimum place to regulate baby's body temperature, but vernix, with its thick, waxy coating, also helps insulate the baby.

- Birth can be a traumatic or stressful time for a baby. The vernix acts as a lubricant in the vaginal canal and decreases friction during delivery. Vernix also smells of mama, which provides comfort and bonding post birth.

ↄ

When the baby is born the vernix may be thick and noticeable, or so thin that it's only in the creases of the skin. Babies born via C-section have more, as it hasn't been rubbed off during delivery through the vaginal canal. Babies born after 27 weeks, but earlier than full gestation retain more, and early preemies (pre-27 weeks), full-term babies, and those born after 40 weeks will have less.

The immune proteins found in the vernix and amniotic fluid are similar to the ones found in breastmilk. During the end of pregnancy, the vernix thins, and some of it sheds into the amniotic fluid that the baby is now breathing. This antimicrobial, peptide-rich mixture enters the baby's lungs and gastro-intestinal tract and helps prepare the digestive tract for the similar peptides found in breastmilk. This process gets the baby's body ready for the transition to the outside world by prepping and nourishing their digestive systems.

As soon as the baby is born, mom and baby need skin-on-skin bonding time on the mother's chest—a great time to massage the vernix into baby's skin gently.

LEAVE IT ON

Care providers may try wiping the vernix off right away after the birth (usually with a towel). Let them know beforehand to keep it on, and remind them if need be. If desired, blood, amniotic fluid, and vaginal secretions can be gently wiped off of the baby, without disturbing the vernix much. Because it is antibacterial and antimicrobial, vernix can help prevent infection of the vaginal canal as the baby passes through. It has superior wound healing properties and even been shown to help perineal tears heal better. Gently rub it in.

WHEN TO GIVE BABY'S FIRST BATH?

The majority of the vernix is absorbed within the first day but doesn't fully absorb until day 5 or 6, so best to wait until then. Gently wipe off any blood, spit-up, or feces with warm water.

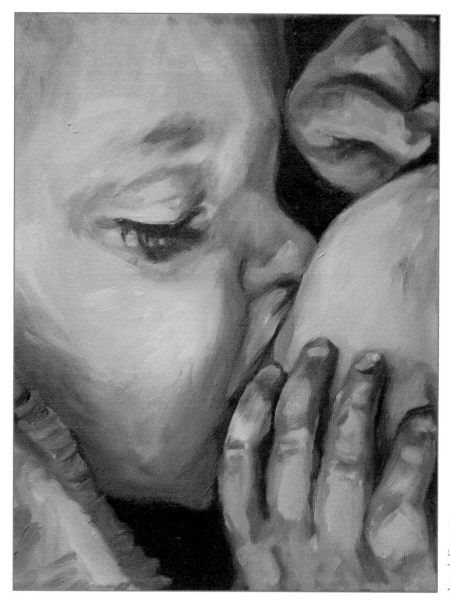

CHAPTER 17:
BREASTFEEDING

"A newborn baby has only three demands. They are: warmth in the arms of its mother, food from her breasts, and security in the knowledge of her presence. Breastfeeding satisfies all three."
- GRANTLY DICK-READ

"People need to understand that when they're deciding between breast milk and formula, they're not deciding between Coke and Pepsi.... They're choosing between a live, pure substance and a dead substance made with the cheapest oils available."
- CHELE MARMET

"In modern consumer society, the attack on mother-child eroticism took its total form; breastfeeding was proscribed and the breasts reserved for the husband's fetishistic delectation. At the same time, babies were segregated, put into cold beds alone and not picked up if they cried."
- GERMAINE GREER

ONE OF THE MOST astonishing aspects of breastfeeding for me was to be down the road from our home, teaching a class, and the tingling, pins and needles-type sensation would arise in my breasts, as the milk was released into the ducts. This is the "let-down reflex" and also occurs when the baby has begun sucking, as the nerves in the breast are stimulated.

The World Health Organization recommends exclusive breastfeeding (no other fluids or solids) for six months, and then continued breastfeeding combined with solid foods for 12–24 months, or as long as mother and baby desire. The American Academy of Pediatrics recommends breastfeeding a baby for the first 12 months. Ayurvedic physician Dr. Subhedar offers this wise perspective: "The best life insurance for your baby is mother's milk and daily oil massage."

The advantages and disadvantages of breastfeeding have been debated for many years. The frequency of breastfeeding in the United States and other highly developed nations of the world diminished significantly from the 1950s through the 1970s. However, with the emphasis on natural foods in the later 1970s, there was resurgence in breastfeeding. The reawakening to the benefits of breastfeeding has been heightened by the devastating effects of attempts to switch from breastfeeding to formula feeding in developing nations. The lack of proper means for sterilization and the fact that many substances important to an infant's resistance to infection are missing from formulas resulted in significant increases in early infant mortality in these countries. A renewed interest in the scientific investigation of human milk has further revealed its many unique properties.

NUTRITION & GROWTH

As a breastfeeding mother, the quality of digestion and nutrition is essential for the quantity and quality of milk. Make sure to drink a lot of water and eat! You may find the appetite to be greater when breastfeeding than when pregnant. Also, continue taking a prenatal vitamin, and get plenty of oils, as the most rapid brain growth occurs during the first year of life, with the infant's brain tripling in size by the first birthday. During this stage of rapid central nervous system growth, the brain uses sixty percent of the total energy consumed by the infant. Fats are a major component of the brain cell membrane and the myelin sheath around each nerve (the brain is around 60% fat). So, it makes sense that getting enough fat can greatly effect brain development and performance.

Mother Nature knows how important fat is for babies; 50% of the calories in mother's milk are fat. During breastfeeding, a baby pulls around 11g of essential fatty acids from the mother daily. Depletion of Omegas 3 and 6 could contribute to women experiencing postnatal depression, stretch marks, fibromyalgia and chronic fatigue amongst other symptoms. A recent review of 75 scientific studies investigating the risk factors for postnatal depression found that women who are at risk could be at even higher risk if their Omega 3 levels are lowered. An outstanding oil to take is called Udo's Oil, using a 3-6-9 blend. This is based on the ideal 2:1:1 ratio of Omega fatty acids, and is made with organic flax, sesame and sunflower seed oils

Brain imaging studies by researchers at Brown University in Providence, Rhode Island, have found that kids who were breastfed exclusively for at least three months had 20 to 30% more white matter. This specific type of brain tissue is rich in myelin, a fatty substance that insulates nerve fibers and speeds up the electrical signals within the brain. The extra white matter growth was seen in areas of the brain associated with language, emotional function, and cognition.

THREE PHASES OF BREASTMILK

The 3 phases of breast milk are: colostrum, transitional milk, and mature milk. A woman's breasts start getting ready to make milk when she becomes pregnant. Breast changes are caused by hormones, which cause the milk ducts and glandular tissue to grow and increase in size. The breasts start to make the first milk, colostrum, in the second trimester. Colostrum is thick, clear to yellow in color, high in protein, and low in fat and sugar. The protein content is three times higher than mature milk, because it is rich in the antibodies being passed from the mother. These antibodies protect the baby and act as a natural laxative, helping baby pass the first stool, called meconium. Once baby and the placenta are delivered, the body starts to make more milk. The milk will change and increase in quantity about 48 to 72 hours after giving birth. As mature milk comes in, the breasts may become very full and feel tender. Continuing to breastfeed every 2 to 3 hours for a minimum of eight feedings a day will help support a good supply.

When starting to breastfeed, the first milk the baby receives is called foremilk. It is thin and watery with a light blue tinge. Foremilk is largely water needed to satisfy your baby's thirst. Hind-milk is released after several minutes of nursing. It is similar in texture to cream and has the highest concentration of fat. The hind-milk has a relaxing effect on the baby. Hind-milk helps the baby feel satisfied and gain weight. Feed a baby until you see a sleepy, satisfied look on their face.

THE HORMONES OF LACTATION

The complex physiology of breastfeeding includes a delicate balance of hormones. There are four hormones that help breasts make milk: estrogen, progesterone, prolactin and oxytocin. The mother's body naturally knows how to adjust the level of these hormones to help the breasts make milk. Oxytocin releases milk from the breasts. When the baby (or breast pump) begins to suck and draw the nipple into her/his mouth, this hormone is released. This release causes milk to be squeezed out of the alveoli (glandular tissue), into the ducts and out of the nipple, into the baby's mouth. This process is called "letdown" or milk ejection reflex (MER).

FACTS ABOUT BREASTFEEDING

1. The metabolic energy needed to breastfeed a baby each day is the amount you'd use to walk seven miles. To use up this many calories, a formula feeding mother would have to swim at least 30 laps in a pool or bicycle uphill for an hour daily.
2. Producing breast milk consumes 25% of the body's energy; the brain only uses 20% by comparison.
3. Newborns held skin-to-skin in the first hour or two after birth may push their way toward mom's breast and start feeding on their own.
4. Human milk is sold on the Internet for $4 per ounce. That's about 262 times the price of oil.
5. Almost three-quarters of moms produce more milk with their right breast (and it has nothing to do with being right-handed).
6. On average, babies remove 67% of the milk mama has available— they eat until fullness, not until the breast is emptied.
7. Breastfed babies can basically pick their moms out of a lineup based on smell alone.
8. Breast milk sprays out of many holes, not just one. The exact number varies from mom to mom.
9. Each nipple has 15 to 20 openings for milk to flow.
10. The amount of breast milk a mom produces has nothing to do with her breast size.
11. Most women with breast implants or reduction are still able to breastfeed.
12. The small bumps on the areola are called Montgomery glands. They produce a natural oily secretion that cleans, lubricates, and protects the nipple during pregnancy and breastfeeding. This oil contains an enzyme that kills bacteria and makes breast creams unnecessary.

Use only water to clean your breasts. Soaps, lotions or alcohol might remove this protective oil, and may not be appetizing or smell good to baby. They want to smell the natural you!

13. Nursing baby triggers the release of the hormone oxytocin, which relaxes you and baby both.

14. US breastfeeding rates were lowest in the late 1960s and early 1970s, when only 20–25% of mothers breastfed.

15. In 2015, 83.2% of US babies were breastfed. However, despite the recommendation to breastfeed exclusively for about the first 6 months, less than 50% of infants were exclusively breastfed through 3 months and about 25% were exclusively breastfed through 6 months.

COW'S MILK FOR CHILDREN?

World-renowned author Benjamin Spock, who wrote the popular book *Baby and Healthcare* a #1 bestseller, in his final edition, before he passed away, issued an apology for ever having recommended cow's milk for children and babies. We are the only species who drink the milk of another species, and well past infancy. In 2002, after being vegetarian for years, I decided to no longer drink the milk or eat the eggs of animals, one reason being that I didn't want to participate in the cruelty of taking milk from the mother cow, which is meant for her baby. In this process, a male bull is aroused by a human hand for their erection and collection of their sperm (bestiality). The sperm is then used to violently impregnate the mother cow, by a human being shoving a metal sperm gun into her vagina without her consent (rape). Immediately after the birth, the calf is taken away (theft), and the mom will never see her baby again. In this anguish, while lactating and grieving the loss of her baby, the mom is hooked up to a milking machine, which is painful and pulls out much more milk than the baby naturally would. Soon after, she is impregnated again. After about 4 years of this torture, she is considered "spent" or "downed" and slaughtered for her flesh, which becomes cheap meat. Her skin likely becomes a purse, belt, or shoes.

The animals eaten and used on a mass scale in the world—cows, chickens, pigs, fish—are babies and toddlers. They are killed at four years old or less. Most of them don't get to see the opposite sex, get to have sex, or enjoy their babies. Taking away these fundamental rights of other species takes away a part of our self, our innocence, and our inner happiness and freedom. One of these facts was reason enough for me to drink milk made from nuts or beans or seeds or coconut. instead.

TYPES OF MILK

- almond
- soy
- coconut
- hemp

- cashew
- rice
- oat
- quinoa

- flax
- potato
- sunflower, etc.

THE AMERICAN ACADEMY OF PEDIATRICS RECOMMENDS BREASTFEEDING

"Human milk is species-specific, and all substitute feeding preparations differ markedly from it, making human milk uniquely superior for infant feeding. Exclusive breastfeeding is the reference or normative model against which all alternative-feeding methods must be measured with regard to growth, health, development, and all other short- and long-term outcomes. In addition, human milk-fed premature infants receive significant benefits with respect to host protection and improved developmental outcomes compared with formula-fed premature infants... Pediatricians and parents should be aware that exclusive breastfeeding is sufficient to support optimal growth and development for approximately the first 6 months of life and provides continuing protection against diarrhea and respiratory tract infection. Breastfeeding should be continued for at least the first year of life and beyond for as long as mutually desired by mother and child." – *A.A.P.*
Breastfeeding Policy Statement: Breastfeeding and the Use of Human Milk Pediatrics Vol. 115 No. 2 February 2005

COLOSSAL BENEFITS OF BREASTFEEDING

1. Breastfeeding satisfies baby's emotional needs and increases bonding between mother and baby. Breast milk provides natural pain relief for baby.

2. Human milk boosts a baby's immune system—helping fight viral, bacterial, and parasitic infections, including: respiratory tract infections, gut infections, ear infections, bacterial meningitis, pneumonia, urinary tract infections, infant diarrhea, common colds and flus, eye infections.

3. Reduces risk of disease later in life, including: Type I and II diabetes, Hodgkin's disease, leukemia, obesity, high blood pressure, high cholesterol levels, Crohn's disease (intestinal disorder), ulcerative colitis, asthma, eczema, Celiac disease, Inflammatory, intestinal tissue damage, bowel disease, osteoporosis, rheumatoid arthritis.

4. Suckling optimizes hand-to-eye coordination, facilitates proper dental and jaw development, and better speech development. Breastfeeding reduces tooth decay and baby's risk of cavities later on.

5. Saves a family approximately $2000–$4000 yearly. Breast milk is free, always ready, the perfect temperature, and the right proportions of fat, carbohydrates, and protein. It is more digestible than formula, and fresh milk is never contaminated with bacteria. Less equipment to buy, maintain and store, less waste producing packaging, bottles to carry around, worry about which brand is best, adding contaminated water to the powder, etc.

6. Can help mothers return to their pre-baby weight. It takes 1000 calories a day on average to produce breast milk. Women are advised to consume an extra 500 calories a day, and the body dips into reserves it built up in pregnancy to make the rest (it's important to consume those extra calories or the body actually goes into "starvation mode" and holds onto the reserves).

7. Milk can change day to day—for example, water content may increase during times of hot weather and baby-sickness to provide extra hydration.

8. Human milk contains substances that promote sleep and calmness in babies.

9. Breastfed infants are at lower risk for sudden infant death syndrome.

10. Mama's breasts can detect even a one-degree fluctuation in baby's body temperature and adjust accordingly to heat up or cool down baby as needed. This is one reason skin-to-skin contact in the early days is so crucial.

11. Breastfeeding mamas sleep an average of 45 minutes more a night, compared to those who formula feed.
12. During breastfeeding, antibodies and other germ-fighting factors pass from a mother to her baby and strengthen the immune system.
13. Cow's milk is designed for baby cows, and is an intestinal irritant for humans. Breast milk contains to genetically engineered materials and no synthetic growth hormones. Breastfed babies get fewer stomach infections, and have less chance of getting eczema.
14. Breast milk aids in the proper development of a baby's gastrointestinal tract.
15. Formula-fed babies are more at risk for obesity and being overweight in later life. Formula feeding increases children's risk of developing diabetes. Formula feeding increases baby's risk of otitis media (ear infections). Formula feeding increases chances of baby developing allergies. Formula costs the government (and taxpayers) millions of dollars.

BREASTFEEDING BENEFITS FOR MOTHER

Most often, the benefits for the baby are praised, and those of the mother are overlooked. The spiritual, physiological, and physical gains for the mother are significant, and lactation provides both short-term and long-term benefits.

Immediately following birth, repeated sucking of the baby releases oxytocin from the mother's pituitary gland. The oxytocin signals the breasts to release milk to the baby and produces uterine contractions, which prevent postpartum hemorrhage and promote uterine involution, or the return to a non-pregnant state.

As long as a mother breastfeeds without substituting formula, foods, or pacifiers, the return of her moon cycles is delayed for many months to years, which conserves iron in the mother's body and can provide natural spacing of pregnancies. Bottle-feeding mothers typically get their cycles back within six to eight weeks. "The amount of iron a mother's body uses in milk production is much less than the amount she would lose from menstrual bleeding. The net effect is a decreased risk of iron-deficiency anemia in the breastfeeding mother. The longer the mother nurses and keeps her periods at bay, the stronger this effect." (Institute of Medicine, 1991).

LONG TERM BENEFITS FOR MOTHERS

- Breastfeeding reduces risk factors for three of the most serious diseases for women: heart disease, osteoporosis, and female cancers (ovarian, breast, and endometrial cancer).
- Heart attacks are the leading cause of death in women. The optimal weight loss, improved blood sugar control, and good cholesterol provided by breastfeeding lower the risk of heart problems.
- Breastfeeding helps decrease insulin requirements in diabetic mothers.
- Because women lose calcium while lactating, some health professionals have mistakenly assumed an increased risk of osteoporosis for women who breastfeed; however, studies have shown that after the child has weaned, breastfeeding mothers' bone density returns to pre-pregnancy or even higher levels, resulting in stronger bones and reduced risk of osteoporosis.
- Ovarian and uterine cancers have been found to be more common in women who did not breastfeed. This may be due to the repeated ovulatory cycles and exposure to higher levels of estrogen from not breastfeeding.

BREASTFEEDING TIPS

Nurse, Nurse, and Nurse Again!
The more baby nurses, the more milk the body makes. Don't follow a strict schedule. Nurse your baby whenever she/he is hungry, for as long as they want, especially in the first few weeks of establishing your supply, and offer the other breast after the first.

Avoid supplementary bottles and pacifiers.
This encourages baby to meet all of her/his sucking needs at the breasts and will help increase milk supply. Pacifiers and bottles can create nipple confusion and baby may begin refusing the breast.

Get adequate rest & avoid stress.
Lack of sleep and stress is rough on your milk production. Spend some days doing very little other than relaxing with baby, resting, eating, and nursing.

(Of course, this is easier with a first baby than when you have older children who also need your attention.)

Massage the breasts.
Can help to boost the volume and fat content of milk. When the baby is "comfort nursing" (calming and soothing herself more than drinking), massage your breast near the chest and then a little farther toward the nipple, and wait for baby to take a couple of swallows. Then massage another area of the same breast, and wait for more swallows.

Drink when baby drinks!
Hydration will help keep the milk coming!

DISCOMFORT

It is not unusual for infant discomfort to occur anywhere in the first 12 weeks of the babies' life. There may be a week or so where the baby is "fussy" for about 2 hours or so per day in the late afternoon or evening. My child did this around 7pm–9pm each night for 6 days when he was an infant. One night a walk in the sling worked, another night having him stare at a fan helped for about 10 minutes, another night singing helped for a little while, etc. Some parents tout the sound of a vacuum cleaner in this time. Gentle bouncing, rocking, keeping them in your arms, and compassionate care can help soothe them. These infants are usually not fussy due to hunger or a wet/dirty diaper. Usually the baby will take their longest stretch of sleep after this time.

During this period, they may want the breast often, seem dissatisfied with feedings and even reject or cry at the breast. This may make the mother feel like something is wrong with her milk, or that the baby isn't satisfied or happy. With the frustration, the parents may "cave" and offer a bottle of expressed breast milk or formula. The baby will guzzle it down, fall fast asleep, and then the parents chalk it up to the idea that baby wasn't getting enough milk. So then they give the baby bottles or formula, which in turn causes a true low milk supply in the mother. Kathy S. Kuhn RN BSN IBCLC and lactation consultant for Parentsplace.com explains it best as to what happens when baby is offered a bottle and guzzles it down:

"When the bottle goes in the baby's mouth the mouth fills with milk, the baby is obligated to swallow and the action of swallowing initiates another suck. The suck again fills the mouth and the cycle repeats, giving an appearance of the baby "gulping the bottle down hungrily. What has really happened is the baby has by coincidence come to the natural conclusion of the fussy spell (most parents give the bottle as a last resort which means the fussiness has been going on for awhile) and/or the baby has withdrawn because "gulping" down the bottle was actually stressful and NOT what the baby wanted but she could not stop the flow, so exhausted, she falls asleep. So don't offer bottles during any fussy time."

BREAST MILK SUPPLY

Often, mothers think that their milk supply is low when it really isn't. If your baby is gaining weight on breast milk alone, then there is no problem. If you aren't sure about weight gain, so long as baby has an adequate number of wet and soiled diapers then the following things do NOT mean that you have a low milk supply: *(From Kelly Bonyata, BS, IBCLC, kellymom.com)*

- The baby nurses frequently. Breast milk is digested quickly (usually in 1.5–2 hours), so breastfed babies need to eat more often than formula-fed babies. Many babies need continuous contact with mom in order to feel safe, and may want to suck. All normal. You cannot spoil the baby by meeting these needs.
- The baby suddenly increases the frequency and/or length of nursing. This is likely a growth spurt. Don't offer baby supplements when this happens, as supplementing informs the body that the baby doesn't need the extra milk, and supply decreases.
- The baby doesn't nurse as long as before. As babies grow, they become more efficient at extracting milk.
- The baby guzzles down a bottle of formula or expressed milk after nursing. Many babies will willingly take a bottle even after they have a full feeding at the breast. (see above explanation)
- The breasts don't leak milk, or only leak a little, or seem softer. These things are normal once your milk supply has adjusted to your baby's needs.

- You never feel a let-down sensation, or it doesn't seem as strong as before. This has nothing to do with milk supply.
- There is very little or no milk when you pump. The amount of milk that you can pump is not an accurate measure of your milk supply. Some women who have abundant milk supplies are unable to get any milk when they pump. In addition, it is normal for pumping output to decrease over time.

TO ENSURE/BOOST SUPPLY TRY:

Water, oats, Mother's Milk tea, nuts, ginger, fenugreek seed, blessed thistle herb. Some research shows that garlic, onions, and mint make breast milk taste different, so your baby may suckle more, and in turn, you make more milk. Make sure that baby is nursing efficiently.

- Nurse frequently and for as long as your baby is actively nursing.
- Take a nursing vacation. Lay in bed all day with baby and let them suckle.
- Offer both sides at each feeding.
- Switch nurse. Alternate breasts multiple times during a feeding.
- Give baby only breast milk.
- Take care of mom.
- Avoid pacifiers and bottles when possible.

PACIFIERS

Babies have a need to suck, because nature designs it that they suck on a nipple for food. Pacifiers are designed after the breast. The baby receives both food and comfort from sucking at the breast. Pacifiers can impede breast-feeding and create early weaning, because the baby is getting their sucking needs met through the pacifier instead. Oftentimes, a baby is given a pacifier more so to pacify the parents than the child. The old adage "children should be seen and not heard," comes to mind. I've seen it many times-as soon as a baby begins to cry, a parent inserts a pacifier into the mouth.

Babies cry to express themselves, just like any person at any age. If every time you wanted to cry, someone plugged your mouth with a rubber nipple, you would likely begin to suppress your feelings and your voice, feeling like no one wants to hear you. I also think about wanting an apple or a lollipop, and then someone giving me a fake one instead of the real thing. A child may be crying because there is a need not being met, or they need soothing in the form of your attention, hugging, singing, rocking, a change of environment, sleep, or they just want to suck on a real nipple.

As the Jan Hunt says, "It is the parents' responsibility to meet their baby's needs for nurturing, security, and love, not the baby's responsibility to meet his parents' need for peace and solitude. Ignoring a baby's crying is like using earplugs to stop the distressing noise of a smoke detector. The sound of a smoke detector is meant to alert us to a serious matter that requires a response—and so is the cry of a baby. As Jean Liedloff wrote in *The Continuum Concept*, "a baby's cry is precisely as serious as it sounds."

GOOD TO KNOW:
- Pacifiers can cause nipple confusion, leading to lack of weight gain for baby, and sore nipples for mother.
- Pacifier use might reduce the baby's frequency or duration of feeds (newborns should be nursing at least 8 to 12 times a day).
- Pacifiers can lead to oral yeast (thrush), which can be transferred to mom's nipples.
- Prolonged pacifier use might result in teeth misalignment, speech problems, and soft palate shaping.
- Studies have proven a link between pacifier use and more ear infections.
- Latex may cause an allergic reaction.

SOME CHALLENGES THAT MAY HINDER BREASTFEEDING

For newborns: prematurity, jaundice, reflux, colic, tongue or mouth malformations.

For mothers: anemia, poor nutrition, sleep deprivation, inverted nipples, severe engorgement or mastitis, and of course no maternal leave from work.

～

Latch-on pain is normal for the first couple of weeks, and should last less than a minute with each feeding. If breastfeeding hurts during feedings, or the nipples and/or breasts are sore, there are lactation consultants who can help. Often, it's a matter of improper latch/technique, but sometimes pain can mean there's an infection. Make sure baby flanges the lips and covers the areola when sucking.

If the baby is dehydrated, not gaining weight or is losing weight, it is possible that a medical condition can cause this. If supplementing is medically necessary, the best thing to supplement with is your own pumped milk. If you are concerned about your milk supply, get in touch with a trained breastfeeding counselor or a board certified lactation consultant.

LACTATION CONSULTANTS

Sometimes a mother needs assistance with breastfeeding from another woman, and lactation consultants can do just that; latching, sore nipples, breast engorgement, and low milk supply are issues they can address. Lactation consultants are trained to assist mothers in preventing and solving breastfeeding difficulties, and commonly work in hospitals, physician or midwife practices, public health programs, and private practice. In the United States, they are often nurses, midwives, nurse practitioners, doulas and dieticians who have obtained additional certification, which includes: completing required health science courses, 90 hours of didactic learning in lactation, clinical experience, and passing a certification exam. In maternity hospitals, there is about one per every 15 postpartum mothers. The U.S. Surgeon General recommends that all communities ensure access to services provided by lactation consultants. Evidence shows that lactation consultants and counselors increased the number of women initiating breastfeeding.

LA LECHE LEAGUE

La Leche League was founded in 1958, and their mission is to help mothers worldwide to breastfeed through mother-to-mother support, encouragement, information, and education, as well as to promote a better understanding of breastfeeding as an important element in the healthy development of the baby and mother.

BASIC PHILOSOPHY OF LA LECHE LEAGUE:
- Mothering through breastfeeding is the most natural and effective way of understanding and satisfying the needs of the baby.

- Mother and baby need to be together early and often to establish a satisfying relationship and an adequate milk supply.
- In the early years, the baby has an intense need to be with his mother, which is as basic as his need for food.
- Human milk is the natural food for babies, uniquely meeting their changing needs.
- For the healthy, full-term baby, breast milk is the only food necessary until the baby shows signs of needing solids, about the middle of the first year after birth.
- Ideally the breastfeeding relationship will continue until the baby outgrows the need.
- Alert and active participation by the mother in childbirth helps in getting breastfeeding off to a good start.
- Breastfeeding is enhanced and the nursing couple sustained by the loving support, help, and companionship of the baby's father. A father's unique relationship with his baby is an important element in the child's development from early infancy.
- Good nutrition means eating a well-balanced and varied diet of foods in as close to their natural state as possible.
- From infancy on, children need loving guidance, which reflects acceptance of their capabilities and sensitivity to their feelings.

WHAT'S IN IT?

FORMULA

Water, Carbohydrates, Lactose, Corn, maltodextrin, Protein, Partially hydrolyzed reduced minerals, whey protein concentrate (from cow's milk), Fats, Palm olein, Soybean oil, Coconut oil, High oleic safflower oil (or sunflower oil), M. alpina oil (Fungal DHA), C.cohnii oil (Algal ARA), Minerals, Potassium citrate, Potassium phosphate, Calcium chloride, Tricalcium phosphate, Sodium citrate, Magnesium chloride, Ferrous sulphate, Zinc sulphate, Sodium chloride, Copper sulphate, Potassium iodide, Manganese sulphate, Sodium selenite, Vitamins, Sodium ascorbate, Inositol Choline bitartrate, Alpha-Tocopheryl acetate, Niacinamide, Calcium pantothenate, Riboflavin, Vitamin A acetate, Pyridoxine hydrochloride, Thiamine mononitrate, Folic acid, Phylloquinone, Biotin, Vitamin D3, Vitamin B12, Enzyme Trypsin, Amino acid, Taurine, L-Carnitine (a combination of two different amino acids), Nucleotides, Cytidine 5-monophosphate, Disodium uridine 5-monophosphate, Adenosine 5-monophosphate, Disodium guanosine 5-monophosphate, Soy Lecithin.

BREAST MILK

Water Carbohydrates (energy source), Lactose Oligosaccharides (see below), Carboxylic acid, Alpha hydroxy acid, Lactic acid, Proteins (building muscles and bones), Whey protein, Alpha-lactalbumin, HAMLET (Human Alpha-lactalbumin Made Lethal to Tumour cells), Lactoferrin, Many antimicrobial factors, Casein Serum albumin Non-protein, nitrogens, Creatine, Creatinine, Urea, Uric acid, Peptides (see below), Amino Acids (the building blocks of proteins), Alanine, Arginine, Aspartate, Clycine, Cystine, Glutamate, Histidine, Isoleucine, Leucine, Lycine, Methionine, Phenylalanine, Proline, Serine, Taurine Theronine, Tryptophan, Tyrosine, Valine, Carnitine (amino acid compound necessary to make use of fatty acids as an energy source), Nucleotides (chemical compounds that are the structural units of RNA and DNA), 5'-Adenosine monophosphate (5"-AMP), 3':5'-Cyclic adenosine monophosphate (3':5'-cyclic AMP), 5'-Cytidine monophosphate (5'-CMP), Cytidine, diphosphate, choline (CDP choline), Guanosine diphosphate (UDP), Guanosine diphosphate-mannose, 3'- Uridine monophosphate (3'-UMP) 5'-Uridine monophosphate (5'-UMP), Uridine diphosphate (UDP), Uridine diphosphate hexose (UDPH), Uridine diphosphate-N-acetyl-hexosamine (UDPAH), Uridine diphosphoglucuronic acid (UDPGA), Several more novel nucleotides of the UDP type, Fats, Triglycerides, Long-chain polyunsaturated fatty acids, Docosahexaenoic acid (DHA) (important for brain development), Arachidonic acid (AHA) (important for brain development), Linoleic acid Alpha-linolenic acid (ALA), Eicosapentaenoic acid (EPA), Conjugated linoleic acid (Rumenic acid), Free Fatty Acids, Monounsaturated fatty acids, Oleic acid, Palmitoleic acid, Heptadecenoic acid, Saturated fatty acids, Stearic Palmitic acid, Lauric acid, Myristic acid, Phospholipids, Phosphatidylcholine, Phosphatidylethanolamine, Phosphatidylinositol, Lysophosphatidylcholine, Lysophosphatidylethanolamine, Plasmalogens Sphingolipids, Sphingomyelin, Gangliosides, GM1, GM2, GM3, Glucosylceramide, Glycosphingolipids,

Galactosylceramide, Lactosylceramide, Globotriaosylceramide (GB3), Globoside (GB4), Sterols, Squalene, Lanosterol, Dimethylsterol, Methosterol, Lathosterol, Desmosterol, Triacylglycerol, Cholesterol, 7-dehydrocholes-terol, Stigma-and campesterol, 7-ketocholesterol, Sitosterol, β-lathosterol, Vitamin D, metabolites, Steroid hormones, **Vitamins:** Vitamin A, Beta car-otene, Vitamin B6, Vitamin B8 (Inositol), Vitamin B12, Vitamin C, Vitamin D, Vitamin E, a-Tocopherol Vitamin K, Thiamine, Riboflavin, Niacin, Folic acid, Pantothenic acid, Biotin, **Minerals:** Calcium, Sodium, Potassium, Iron, Zinc, Chloride, Phosphorus, Magnesium, Copper, Manganese, Iodine, Selenium, Choline, Sulpher, Chromium, Cobalt, Fluorine, Nickel, Metal, Molybdenum (essential element in many enzymes), Growth Factors (aid in the matura-tion of the intestinal lining), Cytokines interleukin-1β (IL-1β) IL-2 IL-4 IL-6 IL-8 IL-10, Granulocyte-colony stimulating factor (G-CSF), Macrophage-colony stimulating factor (M-CSF), Platelet derived growth factors (PDGF), Vascular endothelial growth factor (VEGF), Hepatocyte growth factor -a (HGF-a), HGF-β, Tumor necrosis factor-a, Interferon-γ, Epithelial growth factor (EGF), Transforming growth factor-a (TGF-a), TGF β1, TGF-β2, Insulin-like growth factor-I (IGF-I) (also known as somatomedin C), Insulin-like growth factor-II, Nerve growth factor (NGF), Erythropoietin, Peptides (combinations of amino acids), HMGF I (Human growth factor), HMGF II, HMGF III, Cholecystokinin (CCK), β-endorphins, Parathyroid hormone (PTH), Parathyroid hormone-re-lated peptide (PTHrP), β-defensin-1, Calcitonin, Gastrin, Motilin, Bombesin (gastric releasing peptide, also known as neuromedin B), Neurotensin, Somatostatin, **Hormones** (chemical messengers that carry signals from one cell, or group of cells, to another via the blood): Cortisol, Triiodothyronine (T3), Thyroxine (T4), Thyroid stimulating hormone (TSH) (also known as thy-rotropin), Thyroid releasing hormone (TRH), Prolactin Oxytocin, Insulin, Corticosterone, Thrombopoietin, Gonadotropin-releasing hormone (GnRH), GRH, Leptin (aids in regulation of food intake), Ghrelin (aids in regulation of food intake), Adiponectin, Feedback inhibitor of lactation (FIL), Eicosanoids, Prostaglandins, (enzymatically derived from fatty acids), PG-E1, PG-E2, PG-F2, Leukotrienes, Thromboxanes, Prostacyclins, Enzymes (catalysts that support chemical reactions in the body), Amylase, Arysulfatase, Catalase, Histaminase, Lipase, Lysozyme, PAF-acetylhydrolase, Phosphatase, Xanthine oxidase, **Antiproteases** (thought to bind themselves to macromolecules such as enzymes and as a result prevent allergic and anaphylactic reactions): a-1-antitrypsin, a-1-antichymotrypsin, **Antimicrobial factors** (used by the immune system to identify and neutralize foreign objects, such as bacteria and viruses): Leukocytes (white blood cells), Phagocytes, Basophils, Neutrophils, Eoisinophils, Macrophages, Lymphocytes B lymphocytes (also known as B cells), T lymphocytes (also known as C cells), sIgA (Secretory immunoglobulin A) (the most important antiinfective factor), IgA2, IgG, IgD, IgM, IgE, Complement C1, Complement C2, Complement C3, Complement C4, Complement C5, Complement C6, Complement C7, Complement C8, Complement C9, Glycoproteins, Mucins (attaches to bacteria and viruses to prevent them from clinging to mucousal tissues), Lactadherin, Alpha-lactoglobulin, Alpha-2 macroglobulin, Lewis antigens, Ribonuclease, Haemagglutinin inhibitors, Bifidus Factor (increases growth of Lactobacillus bifidus—a good bacteria), Lactoferrin (binds to iron which prevents harmful bacteria from using the iron to grow), Lactoperoxidase, B12 binding protein (deprives microorganisms of vitamin B12), Fibronectin (makes phagocytes more aggressive, minimizes inflammation, and repairs damage caused by inflammation), Oligosaccharides (more than 200 different kinds!).

Source: bellybelly.com.au/baby/ingredients-in-breast-milk-and-formula/

INTERVIEW WITH LA LECHE LEAGUE LEADER

What got you started in La Leche League?

I lived in New York and had my first child. She was having some challenges with reflux. We had seen several specialists and were getting conflicting advice and conflicting information. I went to a La Leche and was relieved to have support and accurate information and to be able to talk about all the different things I was hearing from the different specialists, and find a plan that worked for us. It was great because I got to meet many new friends and just kept going to see my friends each month. Eventually I trained to be a leader. All of the leaders are moms and volunteer our time.

What does the La Leche League offer?

We have meetings morning and evening. They are all free. We like to call them casual gatherings. They are not classes, but more like a discussion. We have topics such as nutrition, weaning, or starting early feeds. We talk about whatever questions people come with. Most meetings are for mothers only, because women are just getting the hang of breastfeeding, and they want a safe place.

Do you know what percentage of women breastfeed?

I don't know the exact answer, but the CDC has a breast-feeding report at CDC.gov/breastfeeding/reportcard, and they talk about the breastfeeding rates of early days, at six months, and at one year. More women are learning about breastfeeding, and there is more support as people are learning the need for it. The La Leche League is a vital piece of that because their support is vital in keeping that going. A lot of times when moms have a goal of six months or a year, it is not always as easy as they thought when they were pregnant, so when they come up against hurdles, we can support each other.

What are some of the common hurdles that women experience?

For instance, if a mom is going back to work, she might have challenges with daycare. The daycare provider may say you need to send more milk, but if they know how to do pace bottle-feeding, and how to store human milk properly and not waste it, then mom won't feel so discouraged.

Do you help women who have things like mastitis, plugged ducts, infections, etc.? What is your role as a lactation consultant?

As a board certified lactation consultant, my role and scope would be assessment, education, going to houses helping with weight, and talking to pediatricians as well at the parent's request.

Is there a hotline that women can call to reach someone at La Leche League?

There is an 800 line that can be found on LLL.org, but we encourage moms to call local. We can give information about local sources, and if something is out of our scope as La Leche League leaders, we would then refer onwards to lactation consultants, or speech pathologists, or occupational therapists who live in the community.

What are some factors that contribute to a low milk supply?

I would say the number one factor is just needing some information and not understanding how our bodies work. Most women can make more milk by taking out milk. So the more we take out milk from our bodies, the more milk we make. There are a lot of challenges there—if there is separation in the hospital and if somebody isn't helping with education on how to express the milk and get it out while you are being separated. Or if you are being encouraged to schedule or stretch out feedings, rather than feed on demand, then your body isn't being encouraged to give that signal to make milk. There are women who truly do have health challenges, perhaps diabetes or thyroid challenges, or what is called hypoplasia, which is underdeveloped breast tissue, and they don't have enough milk making tissue. Then there are also challenges the baby might have like tongue-tied or low muscle tone or sensory issues or congenital heart issues. But the thing about La Leche League is that we are there to listen to moms and give them resources. Sometimes they can get things done, but sometimes they have to supplement and have to understand that they are making as much as they can. We always ask moms or their families what their goals are for breastfeeding, and then try to help them meet their goals. Sometimes that means redefining their goals for the health of their selves or the babies.

Is there anything else you want to say about La Leche League?

I think an important thing to know is that you are invited to La Leche League. It is a warm and friendly supportive place. In La Leche League we always say, "Take what works for you and leave the rest." We believe parents know their children best, and that they, for the most part, know what is right for their families, and they are there because they care about their kids. So we are not there to tell you what to do or tell you how to run your life. Come while you are pregnant and at anytime. We have moms come who are not experiencing any problems. They come because they want to make friends and meet others who are breastfeeding. You can bring your baby carrier and ask other people to help you learn how to breastfeed in a carrier. You can come because you have questions about baby's teething. In every single meeting I have ever held, we talked about sleep. We talk about sex and we talk about how to handle these things—how do you find time for each other, how do you get to work, how do you get your schedule going for pumping. I think people have outdated information about breastfeeding. I think every week I get a call about medication. There is something called LactMed. One can Google that, and there is a free website where they can look up medications.

Is there any thing else you want to offer in regard to books or movies that you have read or seen that are really helpful?

"The Womanly Art of Breast Feeding" is a fabulous book. I love the eighth edition, because you can read it just a chapter at a time. You don't have to feel like you need to read the whole book. Also, MakingMoreMilk.com's book is called *The Breast Feeding Mother's Guide to Making More Milk*. It has so many different resources, especially if you are a second-time mom who wasn't sure the first time if you were making enough milk and want to try it again; it is really empowering to have that information.

Since our culture is different from other countries, what do you feel about breast-feeding in public?

There are Breast Feeding Coalitions that work on changing the laws, to make sure that breast-feeding in public is legal and supported. There is a website called breastfeedinglaw.com. You can look up the laws by state and by federal law. We don't have a fine for people who harass women when they are breastfeeding in public, but think of how selfish it would be to say, "I can stand and eat in public but the infant can't." It is not illegal in any state to breastfeed in public. But if someone says, "You can't breast feed here," there is no fine or consequence to that person.

ADOPTIVE MOTHERS CAN PRODUCE MILK

Adoptive mothers can breastfeed. This is called induced lactation. Sometimes the adoptive mother already was lactating, but if not, the infant's sucking would bring in a milk supply. Most women who are inducing lactation simply put the infant to breast and practice very frequent breastfeeding and baby-wearing (holding the infant almost constantly in a sling or carrier). Place the baby to breast for 20 minutes, 8 times per day. If an adoptive mother knows in advance when baby will be born, she can start by manually and mechanically stimulating her breasts and nipples using a combination of several minutes of gentle massage and a rental-grade electric breast pump several times per day. Gradually, the woman increases the amount of stimulation until she is pumping for 10 minutes, 8 times during each 24-hour period.

After massage and pumping are begun, some induced lactation efforts begin with physician-prescribed hormones (estrogen and progesterone) that imitate the hormone levels of pregnancy. These medications are withdrawn after a short while, tricking the body into sensing that a baby has been born. The woman may then begin taking another prescribed drug called a galactagogue (a term that means 'a milk stimulating substance'). Although there is no research to confirm effectiveness, some women who don't want to use hormones may use herbal galactagogues such as fenugreek, in addition to pumping and breast massage, to help establish milk production.

The Medela Supplemental Nursing System™ (SNS) allows mother to supplement the baby directly at the breast. The SNS™ is a necklace-like device filled with formula. Thin silicone feeding tubes are taped to the nipple, and the baby drinks formula while breastfeeding. This device provides sucking stimulation for the breasts while ensuring that the baby gets enough to eat. Fathers can tape the feeding tube to a finger, and many fathers share that this experience is far more intimate than feeding with a bottle. (medela-breastfeedingus.com)

SOME PROTOCOLS OF INDUCING LACTATION

"The Protocols for Induced Lacation: A Guide for Maximizing Breastmilk Production" by Lenore Goldfarb, B.Comm, B.Sc, IBCLC and Jack Newman, MD, FRCPC, is a guide that came about as a result of Lenore's own experience with induced lactation, derived from protocols published in in *The Ultimate Breastfeeding Book of Answers* by Dr. Jack Newman (Prima Publishing, 2000).

In 1999, Lenore set about trying to find a way to bring in a milk supply for her son who was to be born via gestational surrogacy. She contacted Dr. Newman as soon as she learned that her son was on the way, and together they set upon a journey that enabled Lenore to successfully breastfeed her son, born 2 months prematurely, from his second day of life. Lenore brought in an astonishing 32 ounces of her own milk per day without going through a pregnancy.

The protocols that Newman developed from ongoing research have helped over 250 adoptive, relactating, and intended mothers to bring in substantial milk supplies. Dr. Newman and Lenore expect to continue to refine the protocols as more information becomes available via their research. They are aware of at least 500 other mothers who were successful at inducing lactation. Induced lactation is also called "adoptive breastfeeding." If the mother's physician is not yet comfortable with this journey, a good lactation consultant familiar with induced lactation can be of assistance. The hospital, birthing center, or home where the baby is to be born should be notified verbally and in writing that the adoptive or intended mother is planning to breastfeed.

During pregnancy a woman's body produces increasing amounts of progesterone, estrogen (via the placenta), and prolactin (via the pituitary). These hormones ready the breasts for breastfeeding. Once the pregnancy is completed, progesterone and estrogen levels drop and prolactin levels increase resulting in lactation. Some methods used in their protocol to help stimulate breast milk are the following: special birth control pill, domperidone dosage, using a breast pump, oatmeal, water, fenugreek seed, and blessed thistle herb.

The release of oxytocin coupled with the draining of milk from the breast causes the breast to produce more milk. But not everyone who induces lactation can make a full supply. Some mix feed with bottles or formula and/or donor breast milk. Even if you cannot make enough to exclusively breastfeed your baby, every drop counts! Also, breastfeeding is not just about the milk but about comfort and mothering as well.

౪

*Resources for more information on this are found in the back of this book. Do research and begin 6 months in advance if possible. There is an accelerated protocol as well if it is unknown as to when the adoption may occur.

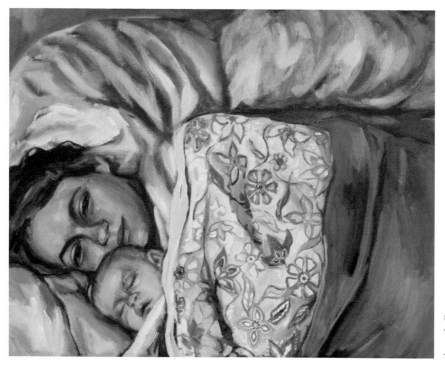

CHAPTER 18: POSTPARTUM

*"New moms need to be taken care of. They need to
feel safe and secure so they can do the most important
thing in the world, care for their new baby."*
— ALISSA SEGERSTEN

*In some cultures, the word for "pregnant mother" is the same
as the word for "new mother," which essentially translates
as Motherbaby: implying that whatever affects the mother also
affects the baby, both before birth and after birth. You can think
of the Motherbaby as a newborn entity who requires a great
deal of care, nourishment, kindness, and support throughout the
slow transition into two separate, distinct beings. She needs to be
fed, held, comforted. She needs sleep, support and safety. Most
of all, a newborn mother should never be left to cry it out alone.
Someone needs to respond to her cries; someone needs to be there
to reach out and say, "I know...it's so hard...it feels impossible,
and yet I know you can do it, because you ARE doing it..."*
— LAURALYN CURTIS

I KNEW THAT SELF-CARE in the postpartum would be most difficult for me, but
also most important. Sleeping, not looking at screens, staying inside, having
meals delivered by friends, eating well, staying hydrated, self-oil massage,
laying low, not talking too much, taking short walks, were all things that I
planned to help me through the newness of having a baby. I wanted it to be
a quiet and peaceful atmosphere. There seemed to be an even more delicate
veil between my inner world and the outer world. Mothers are more sensitive
after birthing.

POSTPARTUM RECOVERY

"Mother the Mother" is a phrase for the experience a woman should have
after giving birth. In the book *The Keys to Postnatal Rejuvenation, 42 days for 42*

years, written by a postpartum doula named Martha Oakes, she writes that choices made in the first six weeks (42 days) after birth influence a woman's health and ability to mother and partner well for the next 42 years. The nature of a mother's unconditional heart makes it easy for her body to serve to the point of stress. Postpartum is not the time for the mother to be hosting friends and family. They are the ones who can serve the mother.

10 KEY ELEMENTS

1. **Mother the Mother:** she needs rest, love, help, & no stress
2. **Be Prepared:** have everything ready, so no need for effort
3. **Nourishment for Mothers:** digestive strength is diminished with childbirth, so it is recommended to eat warm, oily, liquid, moist, delicious, gentle on the digestion, fresh ingredients prepared by a happy cook! Things like coconut milk, sweet fresh fruit, soups, lentils, roasted veggies, etc. …kitchen medicine!
4. **Nourishment for Newborns:** breast milk
5. **Mother's Massage:** massaging sesame oil onto the entire body before bath
6. **Oleation:** edible oils and fats in diet, as well as oil in massage
7. **Infant Massage:** gives baby a sense of their inner self, and helps open up limbs, as well as soothes baby. Excellent for the partner to do as a way for them to touch baby since mother has breastfeeding as a means of bonding. (See technique later in chapter)
8. **Special Needs Herbs:** for teas, tinctures, sitz bath mixture
9. **Essential Oils:** lavender in a diffuser or the like can soothe
10. **Rest & Meditation:** healing of uterus, tissues, bonding

LIST OF THINGS FOR MOTHER

1. Sesame oil (organic, high quality, such as Banyan Botanicals)
2. Organic cotton large menstrual pads (for bleeding after birthing)
3. Cotton balls (to place in the ears to keep wind from entering)
4. Socks or slippers (heat in body is reduced in childbirth, so maintain heat by keeping warm)
5. Warm nightgowns with buttons or snaps up the front (for easy breastfeeding in middle of night, and to stay warm)

6. Mug of tea or water nearby at all times (to keep up hydration and breast milk supply)

7. Non-toxic large pads while vaginal bleeding occurs. To make "padsicles," open the package, squirt some witch hazel on the pad, then roll back up and place back in packaging. Put them all in a freezer bag and in the freezer, so they will be cold. The cold will feel good down there.

8. Peri bottle to fill with warm water to squirt onto vagina after peeing. Toilet paper feels rough after birthing.

9. Herbal blends to facilitate recovery, decrease inflammation, and aid in healing. A sample mixture is yarrow, calendula and chammomile flowers, urva ursi leaf, lavender essential oil, and epsom salt.

   As a Sitz Bath: Add one cup of mixture to six cups of boiling water. Turn off heat and steep for 30 minutes. Pour into your bathwater & enjoy.

   As an Herbal Compress: Boil 2 cups of water and add two tablespoons of the mixture. Let is steep for 5 minutes, then pour into a bowl and soak a washcloth in it for 10 minutes. When warm, gently squeeze out the excess & apply to perineal area for no more than 20 minutes.

   As a Peri-Rinse: Add 4 tablespoons of mixture to 4 cups boiling water. Cool to room temperature. Fill peri-bottle with infusion & gently wash over perineal area to reduce swelling.

   For external use only. Store in a cool place.

PARENTAL LEAVE & TAKING YOUR TIME

This time will never come back again. The baby needs you terribly in these first 6 weeks. The mother needs the closeness of the baby, too.

In the United States, there is a lack of government-sponsored, paid parental leave. There is no federal law requiring private-sector employers to offer paid leave, making the U.S. the only developed country in the world that does not provide this for its citizens. The Family Medical Leave Act (FMLA) gives full-time workers in companies with 50 or more employees up to 12 weeks of unpaid leave. A 2017 survey conducted by the Bureau of Labor Statistics found that only 13% of private-industry employees had access to paid family leave through their employer. Private companies are beginning to expand their policies to provide significant benefits for mothers and fathers, such as Reddit, Amazon, Microsoft, Pinterest, Adobe, Netflix, Etsy, Google, Zillow, IBM. While these changes are great, some feel the government should make laws accordingly, and others think that it should remain up to individual companies.

There is much pressure in America to return to a daily routine, exercise regime, or to go back to work shortly after giving birth. Many mothers decide that taking time to rest isn't possible, thereby depriving themselves of this much needed healing and bonding time for the baby and themselves. But this is the most critical time for mother and baby, who are both psychophysiologically delicate. Daycare costs can be similar to the income at work; therefore, waiting to go back or finding a new job will be worth it. Take this time to stay in, breastfeed baby on demand, gaze into their eyes, rest, rest, rest, and heal from what you have just been through physically, emotionally, mentally. This time is precious and magical and goes by in a blurry flash.

Research has shown that longer maternity leaves, whether paid or unpaid, are associated with a decline in depressive symptoms, a reduction in the likelihood of severe depression, and an improvement in overall maternal health, according to a working paper issued by the National Bureau of Economic Research. One national study of 1,762 mothers found that a one-week increase in maternity leave was associated with a 6% reduction in depressive symptoms from 6 to 24 months after birth. Another found that women who took less than eight weeks of paid leave experienced more depression than those who had longer leaves and were in worse health overall. Mothers who work more than 40 hours a week were more likely to be depressed than those who worked 40 hours or less, according to a study by Child Trends, a research center. Women who go back to work sooner also tend to breastfeed less, which cuts into the benefits that breast milk confers, including better immunity.

POSTPARTUM & YOUR BODY

You will likely experience anywhere from 2 to 6 weeks of vaginal bleeding, and a flow of blood and mucus, called lochia.

CALL YOUR MIDWIFE OR DOCTOR IF YOU EXPERIENCE
ANY OF THE BELOW SYMPTOMS:
- Vaginal flow with unusual smell
- Gushes of bright red blood
- Passing large blood clots (golf ball size or larger)
- Extreme abdominal cramps
- Fever/chills (temperature above 38C or 100F)
- Sharp leg/calf pain
- Dizziness/fainting
- Extreme headaches
- Shortness of breath
- Pain, swelling, discharge from your stitches
- Redness, swelling or drainage from Caesarean incision
- Reddened, swollen sore spot on either breast

ATMOSPHERE

There is a delicateness of the mother and baby after birth. Keep voices, music, televisions, phones, and such low. Refrain from placing a phone or computer on belly or near baby, as there are electromagnetic frequencies absorbed from these devices.

MEAL DELIVERY

MAMAS, DO THIS!!! Do not feel guilty about asking for meals or help. People will be delighted to be of service in this way. It takes a lot of energy to shop, choose what to eat, prepare it, and clean up. When nearing the last few months of my pregnancy, I reached out to my community and to people who care about and support my husband and me through a service called MealBaby.com. Once you register, you include your address, what types of food you choose not to have, like animal flesh, dairy, raw onions or garlic, suggestions for food to bring, best times for drop-off, etc. Then you pick dates, send out an email, and people sign up to bring you food! If you prefer they leave the meal at the door, or if you want them to come in and visit with the baby for a short time, you can specify that too or decide on that day. Another food delivery service is MealTrain. These sites can also be for post-surgery, illness, or death in the family. So, in this way, the family is nourished with food prepared with love by friends and family. The parents can stay indoors, bonding, and resting, which is especially important if it is your first baby. Meals are a beautiful thing to ask for, especially if the parents have gotten enough baby gifts already!

Ask that they bring the food in dishes you can recycle, or if they want them back, to put a piece of tape with their name on the dishes so you can keep track of them.

GOODFOODS FOR POSTPARTUM

If we consider the exertion, blood and fluid loss, and internal logistical shifting of organs, we can easily conclude that postpartum food is most beneficial when it is wholesome and easy on the digestive tract. The focus is on high-calorie, nutrient-dense, easy-to-digest foods that are "warming." In other words, quit the salads for a few weeks and go with cooked food.

- Sweet rice pudding with "warming" spices such as ginger, cinnamon, and cardamom made with white basmati rice
- Broths, Soups, Stews
- Lentils
- Oatmeal
- Yams, Bananas, Apples, Pears
- Tapioca Pudding
- Organic Berries
- Kitchari (mung bean dhal and rice, with optional added spices)
- Healthy fats (avocado, extra virgin olive oil, virgin coconut oil, coconut milk)

AVOID

- Dairy products
- Citrus fruit, especially juices
- Peanuts
- Heavily spiced foods
- Beef (and other meats)
- Raw garlic and onions

- Cruciferous vegetables (broccoli, cauliflower, cabbage)
- Wheat / Gluten
- Refined soy products
- Caffeine (coffee, tea, soda) & Alcohol
- Chocolate
- Prenatal vitamins (the iron may be irritating to baby)

MOXABUSTION

Moxabustion, or moxa, is an ancient element of Chinese Medicine. It involves the use of Artemesia, Chinese mugwort, to heat, nourish, and invigorate the mother's belly following a birth to draw energy and help replenish the substantial loss that took place there. Women love the sensation of deep heat as the herb is burned over their abdomen, and any soreness or prolapsed sensations often disperse after just a few applications. Traditionally, this procedure has been called "mother roasting" and should take place around a week after giving birth.

ANNOUNCEMENT OF BABY

Have a plan to make one major announcement, or have someone else in charge that can do this for you. For instance, parents can let siblings know, and one friend lets all the other friends know, etc. This will help to keep you off the phone and computer and free up time to take care of yourself and baby.

VISITORS IN POSTPARTUM

Place a sign on the door to let people know of the sacred atmosphere.

WELCOME FRIENDS & FAMILY

Little Baby _____ Was Born at _____ on _____

We ask that you please remove your shoes and be quiet upon entering.

Turn off the ringer on your phone.

Wash your hands thoroughly when you come in to ensure cleanliness.

Because this is a precious time, please stay a maximum of 30 minutes, and if possible, any odd jobs around the home you can do are greatly appreciated.

HOME HELP
(sign on fridge perhaps)
- ☐ Laundry load
- ☐ Empty trash can
- ☐ Wash dishes in sink
- ☐ Empty refrigerator of older food
- ☐ Clean toilet and/or sink
- ☐ Wash out delivered food receptacles and set aside
- ☐ Sweep the floor

AFTER BABY & PLACENTA HAVE BOTH BEEN BIRTHED

1. Give mom a sponge bath and apply warm sesame oil all over her body, especially the abdomen. Perform daily oil massage (before getting into the tub) for all 42 days, either by self-massage or scheduling home massage with a trusted and knowledgeable masseuse.

2. Wrap the mom's abdomen with a washable, lightweight cotton cloth, about 4–5 yards by 8–12 inches long. This provides both comfort and support for all the empty spaces to reconnect and reorganize more efficiently.

3. Consider a warm bath for the baby where he/she can "float" unrestricted. Your partner or birth attendant can hold baby with one hand (wrist under the head, thumb, and forefinger around baby's armpit) while you watch. Baby will relax and unfurl their little hands and legs, exploring the water.

4. After baby is dry, apply warm sesame oil on the baby's head, covering the fontanel (soft spot) with some gauze soaked in sesame oil. This is said to be calming, strengthening, and protective.

5. Wrap baby in a cotton or silk cap (advised for the first year) as well as an outer receiving blanket.

6. Drink a lot of fluids—drink when baby drinks. Purified water, Dashamoula Tea, Mother's Milk, Fenugreek, and Red Raspberry Tea (raspberry leaf along with fennel helps the uterus contract), are all great options. This keeps milk supply up and the body hydrated.

Nurse the baby on demand first two weeks, and no less than every two hours after that.

> **DASHAMOULA TEA**
> - 2 tablespoons Dashamoula tea
> - 2 cups water
>
> Boil down to 1/2 cup. Take 1/4 cup warm, twice a day—early in the morning and in the evening. Make fresh daily.

THINGS YOU CAN DO IF FEELINGS OF DEPRESSION CONTINUE AFTER BIRTH

- Breastfeed
- If you experienced any trauma in labor and birth, talk about it with someone
- Get some help with the baby
- Eat placenta if you have saved it/encapsulated it
- Self-massage with sesame or coconut oil
- Give the baby infant massage
- Eat nourishing food, like oatmeal, and drink a lot of water
- Drink Mother's milk tea
- Get fresh air
- Take baths
- Use essential oils like Roman chamomile, lavender, grapefruit, ylang ylang and sandlewood (can be inhaled, used in a diffuser, or on wrists)
- Call a hotline, find others in your area through websites, facebook, etc.
- Ask people for support

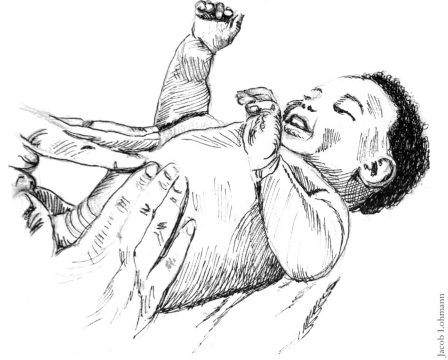

Jacob Lohmann

CHAPTER 19:
INFANT MASSAGE

"Infant massage is one tool we have to help reshape our child's interpretations of the world, to release her pain, grief, and fear, and to open her up to love and joy."
— VIMALA MCCLURE

"I feel like infant massage is a secret that needs to be shared. It has so many benefits and I think our society would ultimately benefit from it with all the other stress we face each day."
— LUANA L, RN

"I heartily endorse the work of Infant Massage USA because the organization understands that touch is not just a good idea, it is a necessary nutrient. I would recommend that you spoil your children with the indulgence of your touch. Perhaps there is nothing quite so personal and intimate as the gift of infant massage, which enriches the parent as well as the baby. Infant massage establishes a tradition of touch that enhances your relationship with your child for years to come."
— PEGGY O'MARA, Mothering

SOME OF THE MOST profound moments between my child and I have come during a massage. Watching him absorb the touch, or looking into each other's eyes, or hearing his "thank you, mommy," after, is so special. Why should we have to wait until we are older and tense or stressed, to pay for and receive a massage? Babies, toddlers, kids, teenagers, can all benefit from massage. Why leave them out? This chapter contains those benefits, as well as the technique. To this day, when I give my child an oil massage, he says with a smile, "Circles on the joints, strokes on the limbs."

It is a superb way to connect for the father/partner, especially in the early years of the child's life, since the mother will have the closeness and skin to skin of breastfeeding. My husband has cried to me several times after giving our child a massage, because it moves him so much.

It is also a splendid opportunity to involve siblings. If there is a two-year-old sister, for example, she can receive a massage from one parent, while the baby receives a massage from the other parent.

Baby massage is an ancient custom in India, the home of Ayurveda, and provides many physical and emotional benefits to the growing child. These include improved bonding between parent and child, development of healthy sleep patterns, and promotion of skin health. Infant massage may continue until the child is old enough to perform self-massage, which can be a life-long practice.

NURTURING THROUGH TOUCH

No matter what age we are, there is the chance of feeling stress. In babies (and into childhood), stressors can come from the birth, hospitalization, pain from medical conditions, shots given, rough handling, absence from the mother, parental stress (preoccupied or angry faces/reactions, rough handling), big changes to routine, over-stimulation, not attending to their needs (such as not feeding when hungry or lack of attention), societal stress, extreme cases such as physical abuse or neglect, and more.

Touch is an integral element of healthy development, our physical and mental well-being, from birth until death. Everyone has the need to be touched. Individuals will have a different relationship for touch, which is impacted by family, culture, experiences, and other factors. Because choices like baby-wearing and co-sleeping are more common in other countries, children in the United States generally receive less touch. We can nurture our children by holding their hand, kissing them, hugging them, cuddling, or placing a hand on their back, shoulder, or arm.

Tiffany Field, head of the Touch Research Institute at the University of Miami's School of Medicine, has done extensive research on the effects of touch, concluding in one 1988 study that massage caused premature infants to gain more weight than their non-massaged peers. Now, more than 100 studies and 350 medical-journal articles later, Field is recognized as the premier expert in, and advocate for, touch research. Studies done with adolescents "supports the notion that less physical affection can contribute to greater aggression. Massage therapy has been effective with violent adolescents, perhaps because the physical stimulation reduced their dopamine levels and increased their serotonin levels. Their aggressive behavior decreased and their empathetic behavior increased." Furthermore, she found that "massage actually increases natural killer cells. Natural killer cells are the front lines of the immune system. They kill viral cells, bacteria cells. We think that the reason that happens is because we're knocking down cortisol levels, the body's culprit stress hormone. Cortisol kills natural killer cells, and so if we can reduce the stress hormones, we can save natural killer cells."

Nurturing means to nourish, protect, support and encourage. It is also defined as the sum of the environmental factors influencing the behavior and traits expressed by an organism. If those factors include touch and eye contact, the atmosphere will reflect this love and attention being received. I recently read that a hug lasting from 6-20 seconds long lowers blood pressure, slows the heart rate, increases oxytocin, and improves mood. If you are new parents, hugging each other for 20 seconds every day can help keep the understanding, peace, and intimacy in the relationship while navigating together.

BENEFITS FOR BABIES

Whether your baby is one day or several years old, massage brings immediate and lasting results. Benefits for infants, babies, and children include the following:

- Provides a special time of communication that fosters love, compassion, and respect
- Improves general well-being
- Provides an intimate time for children to confide in parents
- Improves overall functioning of the gastrointestinal tract
- Promotes relaxation and helps babies self-regulate calm, which reduces crying
- Helps to normalize muscle tone
- Improves circulation
- Enhances immune system function
- Improves midline orientation

- Helps to develop sensory and body awareness
- Enhances neurological development
- Helps baby/child to sleep more in-depth and more soundly
- Helps increase oxygen and nutrient flow to cells. Improves respiration
- Helps improve pain management
- Helps relieve discomfort from teething
- Helps with congestion, gas, and colic
- Enhances release of hormones in the body. The growth hormone can be stimulated, which helps weight gain.
- Reduces levels of cortisol, the stress hormone
- It provides all of the essential indicators of intimate parent-infant bonding and attachment: eye-to-eye, touch, voice, smell, movement, and thermal regulation.
- Stimulates all of the physiological systems. Massage sparks the neurons in their brains to grow and branch out to encompass other neurons.

BENEFITS FOR PARENTS

- Provides all of the essential indicators of intimate parent-infant bonding and attachment: eye-to-eye, touch, voice, smell, movement, and thermal regulation.
- Encourages pre-verbal communication between caregiver and infant
- Helps parents feel more confident and competent in caring for their children
- Helps parents ease their stress if they are a working parent and must be separated from their children for extended periods during the day
- Provides parents with quiet one-on-one time or interactive play with their children
- Creates a regular time of intimacy between parent and child.
- Increases parents' self-esteem by reinforcing and enhancing their skills as parents, and validates their role
- Gives parents the tools for understanding their child's unique rhythms and patterns
- Teaches parents how to read their infants' cues and recognize their states of awareness

- Provides a unique way to interact with the baby if the child is hospitalized. Helps parents feel a more significant part of the healing process
- Daily massage helps parents to unwind and relax
- Provides a positive way for fathers to interact with their infants/children
- Promotes social and emotional development, furthering self-awareness and self-regulation

(above benefits adapted from LovingTouch.com)

COLD PRESSED OILS & UNSCENTED OILS

Use certified organic oil for massage. The traditional massage oil in Ayurveda is sesame, which is warming and nourishing. In general, cold pressed, unscented fruit and vegetable oils such as safflower, sunflower, coconut, almond, jojoba, camellia or macadamia oils can be used for the following reasons:

- They are non-toxic and safe if ingested
- They can contain beneficial nutrients, such as vitamin E, which are good for the skin
- They contain nutrients that help prevent rancidity
- These oils are less slippery when applied, so it's safer to handle your baby after application
- They have no added scent, so infants can still enjoy their parents' natural smell, and are not overwhelmed

ᔐ

Avoid mineral-based oils which are petroleum-derived, may contain toxic contaminants and do not nourish the skin. Essential oils and oils containing perfumes or synthetic ingredients should not be used on babies. Put the oil in a small squeeze bottle to prevent spills. Carry out a patch test with the oil on the baby's arm a day or so before applying to the whole body, to ensure there are no sensitivities. Pour a bit on the palm of your hand, and rub them together. Show your hands to your baby, and verbally ask permission from your baby to give him/her a massage. Receiving approval from your baby is essential before beginning massage.

CONTINUING THE NURTURING TOUCH

The International Association of Infant Massage encourages continuation of massage beyond baby years. They feel that because school-age children experience a lot of stress, massage can help them think more clearly in class, relax during tests, etc. Kids may share about their day during a massage, which allows parents to listen well, with eye-to-eye contact and minimal distractions. Teens may not want to be touched, so it is best when they are open to it. If a child is sick, emotional, tired, they likely want affection—beautifully expressed in a massage. Essential oils can be used, which can further the soothing affect.

GUIDELINES:

- Most practitioners would advocate starting massage after around four weeks of age when the baby has gained strength, and after the navel has healed.
- The palms, rather than the fingertips, should be used to ensure gentle pressure is applied, and the touch should be tender.
- You can massage at any time of the day, but preferably not immediately after feeding or when the baby is hungry or distressed. Make sure baby is calm and relaxed when you perform massage. Many people like to massage their baby in the evening just before bath time to promote a deep relaxing sleep.
- It is important to stop the massage if the baby is not enjoying it.
- Carry out massage in a warm, draught-free place, on the floor or a table, covered with a towel or blanket that can be washed easily. Traditionally, you would sit on the floor with legs straight out, and support the baby between your legs.
- Turn off the television and radio, and talk or sing to your baby while you perform the massage.
- Warm the oil to body temperature by standing the container of massage oil in warm water—test the temperature on the inside of your wrist before applying it to baby's skin.
- Use circles on the joints, strokes on the limbs.

MASSAGE TECHNIQUE

- Begin with the baby lying on her back, and apply the warmed massage oil to the limbs and the whole front of the body in long, sweeping strokes.
- Massage the crown of the head in long circular clockwise strokes.
- Massage around the ears and side of the head in large circular motions.
- Massage both shoulders in circular motions clockwise, and then up and down the arms, then the palm and back of the hands clockwise—massage along the length of each finger.
- Massage the chest very gently.
- Massage the abdomen using a large circular motion around the navel in a clockwise direction
- Massage the hips in a circular, clockwise direction
- Massage up and down the legs, and then the feet, using a clockwise circular motion with the thumb over the soles of the feet.
- Turn the baby over and massage the back of her head in a large circular motion.
- Massage the back very gently up and down in long gentle strokes.
- Massage the buttocks using a circular motion.
- Massage up and down the backs of the legs.
- Place your baby onto her back again and massage the face very gently. Use circular motions over the cheeks. Use a finger to massage along jawbone from the center of chin up to the ear, then long strokes across the forehead from side to side.

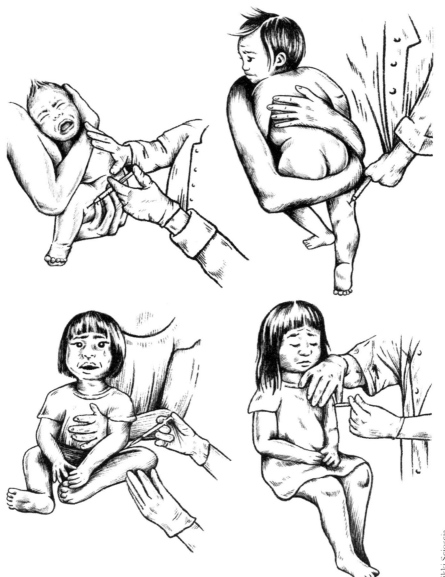

CHAPTER 20: VACCINES

"You inject toxins, you get diseases. Plain and simple. In recent years the vax schedule has catapulted to insane levels since no accountability exists. As has the cancer rate in children. The more vaccines added, the higher the rate of chronically ill children. It's not rocket science."
— LEARNTHERISKS.ORG

"More than 23,000 infants die in the U.S. every year, more than almost all developed countries. Most of these deaths are labeled Sudden Infant Death (SIDs), which is only a label not a real cause of death. Research links SIDs to vaccines."
— LEARNTHERISKS.ORG

"In the United States (and other countries), historical records show that disease mortality declined nearly 90% before the introduction of the vaccine program and routine vaccination programs, according to the Trends in the Health of Americans report. In fact, some of the most prevalent diseases in the early 1900s – including Tuberculosis (TB), Scarlet Fever and Typhoid – followed the same declines WITHOUT ever having a vaccine program. These diseases were nearly eradicated in the U.S. without the population ever having been vaccinated for them."
— LEARNTHERISKS.ORG

THERE ARE FIVE MAJOR manufacturers in the global vaccine market: Merck & Co., Inc., Sanofi, Pfizer Inc., GlaxoSmithKline PLC, and Johnson & Johnson. These companies make millions off of injecting children with chemicals. No one talks about the stories of parents whose child became sick overnight or even died after receiving vaccines. I find it unacceptable that children are used for profit in this way, under the guise, or fear, that they will contract a disease. People will say, "Well, what if your child got rubella from not getting a vaccine?" I say, "And what if I got the vaccine and my child became catatonic or died?" Take a little time to research Dr. Julie Gerberding, who was once director of the CDC, and later the president of Merck. Keep reading, to see that those who do not support the use of vaccines have valid claims and concerns, and consider that those who are deemed "anti-vaccine" may simply be "pro-health."

The best defense against disease is a robust immune system.

Vaccines create temporal (short-term) antibodies only, which is the sole requirement from the FDA to get approval to sell the vaccine. But science has long known that antibodies alone do not create real immunity.

Vaccinations contain many toxic ingredients—some are known to cause cancer and brain damage—which, once injected into the body, go straight to vital organs, bypassing the body's natural line of detox and defense.

Vaccines can contain aluminum, mercury, formaldehyde, antibiotics, yeast, GMOs, animal proteins, animal DNA fragments, and other substances that are potentially dangerous when injected. Usually, vaccines are injected into muscle, where they form a slow-release reservoir intended to stimulate the production of antibodies for some time. The ingredients are not simply flushed out like they might be if taken in as food, and some ingredients such as aluminum and mercury make their way to the brain and accumulate over time. (from learntherisks.org)

⌒

For this chapter, because there is a vast amount of information, science, research, studies, and stories available on this topic, I have chosen to provide you with two things:

1. A list of the ingredients in popular vaccines.
2. A list of educational books and films, with a brief and informative synopsis about each one.

Below is a list of vaccine ingredients per the United States Center for Disease Control website (CDC.gov). It says, "The following table lists substances other than active ingredients (*i.e.,* antigens), shown in the manufacturers' package insert (P.I.) as being contained in the final formulation of each vaccine. Substances used in the manufacture of a vaccine but not listed as contained in the final product (*e.g.*, culture media) can be found in each (P.I.), but are not shown on this table."

VACCINE	INGREDIENTS
Adenovirus	human-diploid fibroblast cell cultures (strain WI-38), Dulbecco's Modified Eagle's Medium, fetal bovine serum, sodium bicarbonate, monosodium glutamate, sucrose, D-mannose, D-fructose, dextrose, human serum albumin, potassium phosphate, plasdone C, anhydrous lactose, microcrystalline cellulose, polacrilin potassium, magnesium stearate, microcrystalline cellulose, magnesium stearate, cellulose acetate phthalate, alcohol, acetone, castor oil, FD&C Yellow #6 aluminum lake dye
Anthrax (Biothrax)	amino acids, vitamins, inorganic salts, sugars, aluminum hydroxide, sodium chloride, benzethonium chloride, formaldehyde
BCG (Tice)	glycerin, asparagine, citric acid, potassium phosphate, magnesium sulfate, iron ammonium citrate, lactose
Cholera (Vaxchora)	casamino acids, yeast extract, mineral salts, anti-foaming agent, ascorbic acid, hydrolyzed casein, sodium chloride, sucrose, dried lactose, sodium bicarbonate, sodium carbonate
DT (Sanofi)	aluminum phosphate, isotonic sodium chloride, formaldehyde, casein, cystine, maltose, uracil, inorganic salts, vitamins, dextrose
DTaP (Daptacel)	aluminum phosphate, formaldehyde, glutaraldehyde, 2-phenoxyethanol, Stainer-Scholte medium, casamino acids, dimethyl-beta-cyclodextrin, Mueller's growth medium, ammonium sulfate, modified Mueller-Millercasamino acid medium without beef heart infusion, 2-phenoxyethanol
DTaP (Infanrix)	Fenton medium containing a bovine extract, modified Latham medium derived from bovine casein, formaldehyde, modified Stainer-Scholte liquid medium, glutaraldehyde, aluminum hydroxide, sodium chloride, polysorbate 80 (Tween80)
DTaP-IPV (Kinrix)	Fenton medium containing a bovine extract, modified Latham medium derived from bovine casein, formaldehyde, modified Stainer-Scholte liquid medium, glutaraldehyde, aluminum hydroxide, VERO cells, a continuous line of monkey kidney cells, Calf serum, lactalbumin hydrolysate, sodium chloride, polysorbate 80 (Tween 80), neomycin sulfate, polymyxinB
DTaP-IPV (Quadracel)	modified Mueller's growth medium, ammonium sulfate, modified Mueller-Miller casamino acid medium without beef heart infusion, formaldehyde, ammonium sulfate aluminum phosphate, Stainer-Scholte medium, casamino acids, dimethyl-beta-cyclodextrin, MRC-5cells, normal human diploid cells, CMRL 1969 medium supplemented with calf serum, Medium 199 without calf serum, 2-phenoxyethanol, polysorbate 80, glutaraldehyde, neomycin, polymyxin B sulfate
DTaP-HepB-IPV (Pediarix)	Fenton medium containing a bovine extract, modified Latham medium derived from bovine casein, formaldehyde, glutaraldehyde, modified Stainer-Scholte liquid medium, VERO cells, a continuous line of monkey kidney cells, calf serum and lactalbumin hydrolysate, aluminum hydroxide, aluminum phosphate, aluminum salts, sodium chloride, polysorbate 80 (Tween 80), neomycin sulfate, polymyxin B, yeast protein.
DTaP-IPV/Hib (Pentacel)	aluminum phosphate, polysorbate 80, sucrose, formaldehyde, glutaraldehyde, bovine serum albumin, 2-phenoxyethanol, neomycin, polymyxin B sulfate, modified Mueller's growth medium, ammonium sulfate, modified Mueller-Miller casamino acid medium without beef heart infusion, Stainer-Scholte medium, casamino acids, dimethyl-beta-cyclodextrin. MRC-5 cells (a line of normal human diploid cells), CMRL 1969 medium supplemented with calf serum, Medium 199 without calf serum, modified Mueller and Miller medium
Hib (ActHIB)	sodium chloride, modified Mueller and Miller medium(the culture medium contains milk-derive draw materials (casein derivatives), formaldehyde, sucrose
Hib (Hiberix)	saline, synthetic medium, formaldehyde, sodium chloride, lactose

VACCINE	INGREDIENTS
Hib (PedvaxHIB)	complex fermentation media, amorphous aluminum hydroxyphosphate sulfate, sodium chloride
Hep A (Havrix)	MRC-5 human diploid cells, formalin, aluminum hydroxide, amino acid supplement, phosphate- buffered saline solution, polysorbate20, neomycin sulfate, aminoglycoside antibiotic
Hep A (Vaqta)	MRC-5 diploid fibroblasts, amorphous aluminum hydroxyphosphate sulfate, non-viral protein, DNA, bovine albumin, formaldehyde, neomycin, sodium borate, sodium chloride
Hep B (Engerix-8)	aluminum hydroxide, yeast protein, sodium chloride, disodium phosphate dihydrate, sodium dihydrogen phosphate dihydrate
Hep B (Recombivax)	soy peptone, dextrose, amino acids, mineral salts, phosphate buffer, formaldehyde, Potassium aluminum sulfate, amorphous aluminum hydroxyphosphate sulfate, yeast protein
Hep B (Heplisav-B)	vitamins and mineral salts, yeast protein, yeast DNA, deoxycholate, phosphorothioate linked oligodeoxynucleotide, phosphate buffered saline, sodium phosphate, dibasic dodecahydrate, monobasic dehydrate, polysorbate 80
Hep NHep B (Twinrix)	MRC-5 human diploid cells, formalin, aluminum phosphate, aluminum hydroxide, amino acids, sodium chloride, phosphate buffer, polysorbate 20, neomycin sulfate, yeast protein
Human Papillomavi, us (HPV) (Gardasil 9)	vitamins, amino acids, mineral salts, carbohydrates, amorphous aluminum hydroxyphosphate sulfate, sodium chloride, L-histidine, polysorbate 80, sodium borate, yeast protein
Influenza (Afluria) Trivalent & Quadrivalent	sodium chloride, monobasic sodium phosphate, dibasic sodium phosphate, monobasic potassium phosphate, potassium chloride, calcium chloride, sodium taurodeoxycholate, ovalbumin, sucrose, neomycin sulfate, polyrnyxin B, beta-propiolactone, thimerosal (multi dose vials)
Influenza (Fluad)	squalene, polysorbate 80, sorbitan trioleate, sodium citrate dehydrate, citric acid monohydrate, neomycin, kanamycin, barium, egg proteins, cetyltrimethylammonium bromide (CTAB), formaldehyde
Influenza (Fluarix) Trivalent & Quadrivalent	octoxynol-10 (TRITONX-100), u-tocopheryl hydrogen succinate, polysorbate 80 (Tween 80), hydrocortisone, gentamicin sulfate, ovalbumin, formaldehyde, sodium deoxycholate, sodium phosphate-buffered isotonic sodium chloride
Influenza (Flublok) Trivalent & Quadrivalent	sodium chloride, monobasic sodium phosphate, dibasic sodium phosphate, polysorbate 20 (Tween 20), baculovirus and Spodoptera frugiperda cell proteins, baculovirus and cellular DNA, Triton X-100, lipids, vitamins, amino acids, mineral salts
Influenza (Flucelvax) Trivalent & Quadrivalent	Madin Darby Canine Kidney (MDCK) cell protein, protein other than HA, MDCK cell DNA, polysorbate 80, cetyltrimethlyammonium bromide, and B-propiolactone
Influenza (Fluvirin)	ovalbumin, formaldehyde, sodium deoxycholate, a-tocopheryl hydrogen succinate, polysorbate 80, thimerosal (multi-dose vials)
Influenza (Flulaval) Trivalent & Quadrivalent	formaldehyde, egg protein, octylphenol ethoxylate (Triton X-100), sodium phosphate-buffered isotonic sodium chloride solution, thimerosal (multi-dose vials), sucrose
Influenza (Fluzone) Quadrivalent	egg protein, octylphenol ethoxylate (Triton X-100), sodium phosphate-buffered isotonic sodium chloride solution, formaldehyde, sucrose
	*above ingredients sourced from FDA.gov

VACCINES	ABORTED FETAL TISSUE IN VACCINES
Hep A/Hep B (Twinrix)	Formalin, yeast protein, aluminum phosphate, aluminum hydroxide, amino acids, phosphate buffer, polysorbate 20, neomycin sulfate, MRC-5 human diploid cells
Hep A (Havrix)	Aluminum hydroxide, amino acid supplement, polysorbate 20, formalin, neomycin sulfate, MRC-5 cellular proteins
MMR (MMR-II)	Medium 199, Mimimum Essential Medium, phosphate, recombinant human albumin, neomycin, sorbitol, hydrolyzed gelatin, chick embryo cell culture, WI-38 human diploid lung fibroblasts

VACCINES	ABORTED FETAL TISSUE IN VACCINES
Varicella (Varivax)	sucrose, phosphate, glutamate, gelatin, monosodium L-glutamate, sodium phosphate monobasic, potassium chloride, EDTA, residual components of MRC-5 cells including DNA and protein, neomycin, fetal bovine serum, human diploid cell cultures (WI-38), embryonic guinea pig cell cultures, human embryonic lung cultures
Zoster (Shingles-Zostavax)	sucrose, hydrolyzed porcine gelatin, monosodium L-glutamate, sodium phosphate dibasic, potassium phosphate monobasic, neomycin, potassium chloride, residual components of MRC-5 cells including DNA and protein bovine calf serum
	*above ingredients sourced from the Center for Disease Control (CDC)

DO YOU KNOW WHAT'S IN A VACCINE?

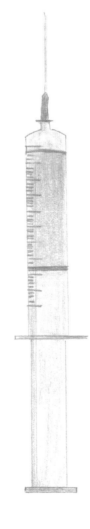

Aluminum
Known to cause brain damage at all doses, linked to Alzheimers Disease, dementia, seizures, autoimmune issues, SIDS, and cancer. This toxin accumulates in the brain and causes more damage with each dose.

Beta-Propiolactone
Known to cause cancer. Suspected gastrointestinal, liver, nerve, and respiratory, skin, and sense organ poison.

Gentamicin Sulphate & Polymyxin B (antibiotics)
Allergic reactions can range from mild to life-threatening.

Genetically Modified Yeast, Animal, Bacteria & Viral DNA
Can be incorporated into the recipient's DNA and cause unknown genetic mutations.

Glutaraldehyde- Poisonous if ingested. Causes birth defects in animals.

Formaldehyde (formalin)
Known to cause cancer in humans. Probable gastrointestinal, liver, respiratory, immune, nerve, and reproductive system poision. Banned from injectables in most European countries.

Polysorbate 80 & 20
Known to cause cancer in animals and linked to numerous autoimmune issues and fertility.

Latex Rubber- Can cause life-threatening allergic reactions.

Human and Animal Cells
Human DNA from aborted babies. Pig blookd, horse blood, rabbit brains, dog kidneys, cow hearts, monkey kidneys, chick embryos, calf serum, sheep blood & more. Linked to childhood leukemia and diabetes.

Mercury (thimerosal)
One of the most toxic substances known. Even if a thermometer breaks, the building is cleared and Hazmat is called. Tiny doses cause damage to the brain, gut, liver, bone marrow, nervous system and/or kidneys. Linked to autoimmune disorders, and neurological disorders like Austism.

Monosodium Glutamate (MSG)
A toxic chemical that is linked to birth defects, developmental delays and infertility. Banned in Europe.

Neomycin Sulphate (antibiotic)
Interferes with vitamin B6 absorption, which can lead to epilepsy and brain damage. Allergic reactions can range from mild to life-threatening.

Phenol/Phenoxyethanol (2-PE)
Used as an anti-freeze. Toxic to all cells and capable of destroying the immune system.

Tri(n) Butylphosphate- Toxic to the kidneys and nervous system.

LearnTheRisk.org

285

BOOKS

Miller's Review of Critical Vaccine Studies

Many people sincerely believe that all vaccines are safe, adverse reactions are rare, and no peer-reviewed scientific studies exist showing that vaccines can cause harm. This book contains summaries of 400 important scientific papers to help parents and researchers enhance their understanding of vaccinations.

Rising From The Dead

This entertaining autobiography tells of one doctor's path through medical school and out into academia, specialty medicine, and practice, having to conform to the system's standards. One day she realized that policy was harming her patients and took a stand.

Saying No To Vaccines: A Resource Guide for All Ages

An in-depth examination by an internationally recognized expert and the first physician to offer documented proof that vaccines compromise the immune system. Dr. Tenpenny substantiates her work with citations directly from the Centers for Disease Control documents and peer-reviewed journals, offering irrefutable facts.

Overdosed America: The Broken Promise of American Medicine

Drawing on his background in statistics, epidemiology, and health policy, John Abramson, M.D., reveals how drug companies have misrepresented statistical evidence and misled doctors. It is an unflinching exposé of American medicine.

Dissolving Illusions: Disease, Vaccines, and The Forgotten History

Provides facts and figures from long-overlooked medical journals, books, newspapers, and other sources, and uses myth-shattering graphs to show that vaccines, antibiotics, and other medical interventions are not responsible for the increase in lifespan and the decline in mortality from infectious diseases.

Selling Sickness: How the World's Biggest Pharmaceutical Companies Are Turning Us All Into Patients

Thirty years ago, the head of Merck, one of the world's largest drug companies, told Fortune magazine that he wanted Merck to be more like chewing gum maker Wrigley's. It had long been his dream to make drugs for healthy people so that Merck could "sell to everyone." Drug companies are systematically working to widen the very boundaries that define illness, and the markets for medication grow ever larger. Mild problems are redefined as serious illness, and common complaints are labeled as medical conditions requiring drug treatments. Runny noses are now allergic rhinitis, PMS has become a psychiatric disorder, and hyperactive children have ADD. Selling Sickness reveals how widening the boundaries of illness and lowering the threshold for treatments is creating millions of new patients and billions in profits.

Vaccine Epidemic: How Corporate Greed, Biased Science, and Coercive Government Threaten Our Human Rights, Our Health, and Our Children

Vaccination is a serious medical intervention that always carries the potential to injure and cause death as well as to prevent disease. Coercive vaccination policies deprive people of free and informed consent—the hallmark of ethical medicine. Americans are increasingly concerned about vaccine safety and the right to make individual, informed choices together with their healthcare practitioners. This book focuses on the debate surrounding individual and parental vaccination choice in the United States.

How to Raise a Healthy Child in Spite of Your Doctor: One of America's Leading Pediatricians Puts Parents Back in Control of Their Children's Health

Dr. Robert Mendelsohn, renowned pediatrician, and author, advises parents on home treatment and diagnosis of colds and flus, childhood illnesses, vision and hearing problems, allergies, and more. Includes a section on picking the right doctor for your child, step-by-step instructions for knowing when to call a doctor, and more.

Vaccines: Are They Really Safe and Effective?
This bestselling immunization handbook (updated 2015 edition) evaluates each vaccine for safety, efficacy, and long-term effects. It contains important, uncensored information, significant studies, several case histories detailing vaccine-induced damage to children, and pinpoints for parents exact conditions that may put their own child at high risk. There are 30 graphs and diagrams and over 900 footnotes and scientific references so that all of the information may be confirmed.

Evidence of Harm: Mercury in Vaccines and the Autism Epidemic: A Medical Controversy
This critical and troubling book reveals the unsung obstacles faced by desperate families who have been opposed by the combined power of the federal government, health agencies, and pharmaceutical giants. From closed meetings of the FDA, CDC, and drug companies, to the mysterious rider inserted into the 2002 Homeland Security Bill that would bar thimerosal litigation, to open hearings held by Congress, this book shows an establishment determined to deny "evidence of harm" that might be connected with thimerosal and mercury in vaccines.

Plague: One Scientist's Intrepid Search for the Truth about Human Retroviruses and Chronic Fatigue Syndrome (ME/CFS), Autism, and Other Diseases
On July 22, 2009, a special meeting was held with twenty-four leading scientists at the National Institutes of Health to discuss early findings that a newly discovered retrovirus was linked to chronic fatigue syndrome, prostate cancer, lymphoma, and eventually neurodevelopmental disorders in children.

Science for Sale: How the U.S. Government Uses Powerful Corporations and Leading Universities to Support Government Policies, Silence Top Scientists, Jeopardize Our Health, and Protect Corporate Profits
The government hires scientists to support its policies; industry hires them to support its business, and universities hire them to bring in grants that are handed out to support government policies and industry practices. The science they create is often only an illusion, designed to deceive; and the scientists they destroy to protect that illusion are often our best.

Vaccination is Not Immunization (4th edition 2015)

The parent's definitive book, a complete vaccine education, meticulously documented with almost 300 references, does not represent special interests. It contains the ingredients of vaccines, vaccine side effects, the dangers of vaccines, autism and vaccines, HPV vaccine, and vaccine cover-ups.

Naturally Healing Autism: The Complete Step By Step Resource Handbook for Parents

The definition of "recovery" is to regain health. If you feel that your child's physical and mental health could improve, then this book is for you. Drug-free recovery is possible. In healing your child's body, you will also enhance abilities such as learning, social adaptability, and self-control. Stages of healing include: repairing the gut, supporting the liver, testing for and treating pathogenic microbes, heavy metal detoxification, brain repair, and support.

The Truth About the Drug Companies: How They Deceive Us and What to Do About It

Dr. Angell proposes a program of vital reforms, which includes restoring impartiality to clinical research and severing the ties between drug companies and medical education. Written with fierce passion and substantiated with in-depth analysis.

Make an Informed Vaccine Decision for the Health of Your Child: A Parent's Guide to Childhood Shots

The current schedule of recommended vaccines is so crowded that doctors give babies several shots during a single office visit—up to eight vaccines all at one time. Vaccines are drugs. How often do we, as adults, take that many drugs at the same time? Would we be more surprised if we did or did not have an adverse reaction? Author Dr. Mayer Eisenstein has practiced medicine, delivered babies, and provided families with preventive healthcare services for over 35 years.

FILMS

Bought: Your Health Now Brought to You by Wall Street
The hidden story behind vaccines, big pharma, and your food. The food, vaccine, drug, insurance, and health industry are a multi-billion dollar enterprise, who are focused more on profits than on human lives. Featuring exclusive interviews with the world's most acclaimed experts in research, medicine, holistic care, and natural health.

The Greater Good
Hear stories of families who have had to deal with the devastating effects from vaccines. Includes differing views of leading authorities on vaccines and vaccine safety, including doctors, scientists, activists and policymakers, as well as the link between vaccines and chronic illnesses such as asthma, allergies, learning disabilities, behavioral problems, autism, unexplained infant death as well as autoimmune diseases such as diabetes, lupus, multiple sclerosis and rheumatoid arthritis. Hear what experts have to say on both sides of the coin.

Injecting Aluminum
In the early 90s, a mysterious muscular disease with symptoms that included severe muscle and joint pain, muscle weakness, fatigue, and fever began to surface among multiple patients in France. A team of doctors and researchers relentlessly studied the patients and eventually discovered that these patients had developed a new disease, called Macrophagic Myofascitis, or MMF, which occurs when the aluminum hydroxide adjuvant from a vaccine remains embedded in the muscle tissue and causes an immune reaction. Aluminum is now known to be neurotoxic and the root cause of many serious illnesses. What the pharmaceutical companies do not make public is that the use of aluminum as a vaccine adjuvant was never rigorously tested before going on the market. The Aluminum adjuvant was only tested for 28 days, on two rabbits, the remains of which have mysteriously disappeared.

Trace Amounts
During the past 20 years, the frequency of autism occurring in children has skyrocketed from 1 in 10,000 to 1 in 68, and the scientific community is no closer to determining a cause. Could a tragedy, which brought one of the

greatest nations to its knees, and stole a generation of children, have been avoided? Watch this film, and you decide.

Autism Yesterday

A documentary that explores an emerging truth many parents are discovering: Autism is a reversible condition through a process known as "biomedical intervention." Through the eyes of five families and their recovering children, Autism Yesterday chronicles heart-wrenching stories of despair, hope, and recovery. This 30-minute documentary puts an extraordinarily controversial topic into the hands of the viewer to decide, through the words of the families and affected children, where the truth lies.

Vaxxed: From Cover-Up to Catastrophe

In 2014, biologist Dr. Brian Hooker received a call from a senior scientist at the U.S. Centers for Disease Control and Prevention (CDC), who led the agency's 2004 study on the Measles-Mumps-Rubella (MMR) vaccine and its link to autism. The scientist confessed that the CDC had omitted crucial data in their final report that revealed a causal relationship between the MMR vaccine and autism. This film examines the evidence behind an appalling cover-up, featuring interviews with pharmaceutical insiders, doctors, politicians, and parents of vaccine-injured children, revealing an alarming deception that has contributed to potentially the most catastrophic epidemic of our lifetime.

Vaxxed II: The People's Truth

In 2016, a media firestorm erupted when Tribeca Film Festival pulled its documentary selection, Vaxxed: From Cover-Up to Catastrophe, amid pressure from pro-pharmaceutical interests. But theatres still showed the film, and the immense volume of parents lining up outside the theaters with vaccine injury stories to share, led producer Polly Tommey to livestream worldwide. She reached millions, and a community that had once been silenced, were empowered to rise up. In this film, you will see interviews of parents and doctors with nothing to gain and everything to lose, as they expose the vaccine injury epidemic and ask the question on parent's minds, "Are vaccines really as safe and effective as we've been told?"

Man Made Epidemic

Filmmaker Natalie Beer sets off on a journey around the world speaking to leading doctors, scientists and families to find out the truth about the autism epidemic and whether or not vaccines have a role to play. The film explores the common misconception that autism is solely genetic and looks into scientists concerns over recent years about environmental factors such as medication and pesticides, which continue to leave our children with physical and neurological damage.

STORY OF RYAN JOHNSON OF NEW HAMPSHIRE

Ryan was a happy, healthy 15-month-old boy. He started walking at 13-months-old and was developing perfectly. He was playful, engaging, and enjoying life. On Friday, October 28th, 2011, Ryan received his routine vaccinations—DTaP, Influenza, HIB, and Pneumococcal.

According to Ryan's mother, he experienced a low-grade fever immediately after the vaccine, and his injection site was tender and inflamed. Twenty-four hours later, he was still very lethargic and no longer actively engaging with anything or anyone, including his family. He slept much longer than usual. She was concerned, but the doctor told her it was a normal reaction.

The day after, the mother took Ryan to daycare. Around midday, while at work, she received a call that Ryan had passed away while napping.

This is not an isolated event.

STORY OF AVIANA PORTER

by her mother Taylor Porter

"Aviana turned four-months-old on May 24, 2017, so it was time for another "well-child visit." I remember crying with Avi when she cried after they injected those vaccinations into her, one nurse on each side. I had never heard her scream so loud in my life, and my heart was broken. The instant they were done, her eyes became heavy. The rest of the day, she was fussier than usual. She was a very happy baby on any other day. She was also very tired and slept more than she usually did.

I went to work as usual a few hours later, so she was with her babysitter until my mom got off of work. I picked Aviana up from my mom's house that night when I got off work around 8:30. They told me she had been a little fussy, was very tired, and not her normal talkative, playful self.

Aviana was usually vocal, cooing, babbling, laughing, and alert. So I chalked up this abnormal behavior to the "normal" reactions to shots because that's what they tell you. They advise not to come in unless the baby's fever is high. I took Aviana home, changed, and fed her. She fell right asleep as she finished her feeding, which was another abnormal for her.

I laid her down around 9:30 or 10, and when I checked on her before I went to bed at 11:30, she was lying on her left side. Aviana had been sleeping through the night for two months, so I didn't think anything of not hearing her throughout the night, because she was a good sleeper. I woke up at 6 am the next morning to get ready for class and went to check on her before I started my routine. Then I peeked in and began to worry.

I ran over to her and found her blue and discolored with bloody mucous fluids coming out of her nose. Her little body was heavy and lifeless, and I knew nothing could be done at this point. Within around 12 hours of receiving her four-month vaccinations, my precious baby was dead.

When EMS arrived, they told me what I knew, but didn't want to hear, which was that there was nothing they could do.

This day will replay over and over again for me for the rest of my life. I had no idea about vaccinations, what was in them, the side effects. I knew NOTHING because they don't truly inform you as a parent. You're just supposed to blindly trust it. I wanted to do what was best for Aviana, which I thought was vaccinating her, and for that reason, she is no longer with me today.

Her autopsy report says "Unknown, undetermined," but there is evidence of it being caused by the vaccines in that report, and I know in my heart that's why."

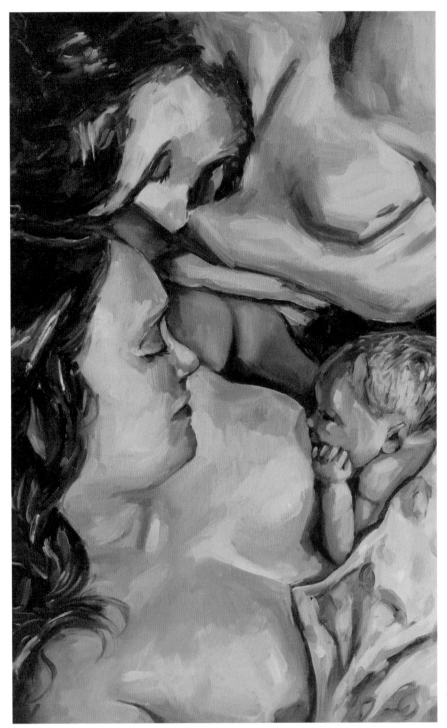

Amanda Greavette

CHAPTER 21:
WHAT TO BUY FOR BABY

I AM GRATEFUL TO have a mother who is an example of practicality and simplicity and has always taught me that a lot of things aren't necessary. "Change the baby on the bed," she said to me. I agreed! "Get a nice blanket." That is about it. Babies want love, closeness, attention, and touch. Get in the bathtub with them and lay them on your legs. All of the money you would spend on so many things…save it for their car, or schooling, or whatever else you can think of. Because most of what you will buy, they grow out of it pretty fast. Which is why you can find a lot of baby consignment!

TOP MATERIAL ESSENTIALS:

- Baby carrier (worn on the body, *i.e.,* Baby Bjorn, Ergo, sling)
- Infant car seat
- Ergonomic baby bouncer
- Warm blanket
- Stroller
- Diapers & Wipes
- Baby nail scissors
- Soft washcloths
- Thermometer
- Cotton hat to cover ears

Baby Bjorn makes a good carrier and bouncy seat. Piyo Piyo makes good scissors. Soft washcloths get in between toes and fingers, as lint gathers in those crevices, and are good for wetting and gently removing anything from around baby's eyes and ears.

NOT ESSENTIAL BUT GREAT TO HAVE:

- Breastfeeding support pillow (*e.g.,* Boppy)
- Snot sucker (*e.g.,* Nose Frida)
- Soft bristle hairbrush

MUST NOT HAVE LIST:

- Diapers with chemicals
- Wipes with chemicals
- Fancy nursery

BABY'S ROOM

There are so many things you can buy to make a room pleasant for baby, but keep in mind that the baby doesn't care what the room looks like—they just want to be held and feel safe and loved. They also want to be with you and sleep near/with you. It's not necessary to buy a changing table, a new lamp, or paint the walls. Change their diapers on the bed! Use a basket to keep diapers in. Hang a couple of shelves or get a pocket hanging wall organizer. A rocking chair is great to have, but you can also rock your body with them in your arms.

DIAPERS

Cloth diaper covers, all-in-ones, and disposables are some options for baby's tushy. A few brands of disposables that are the least toxic for their skin: Bambu, Seventh Generation, & Honest Company.

Organic Clothing for Babies: Burts Bees, Milkbarn, Under the Nile, Hanna Andersson, Pact, Boden, Jazzy, Baby Hero, Finn+Emma, Mini Mioche, & Touched by Nature

DIAPER CREAMS

There are many ointments and creams for diaper rash, but if the diapers and wipes are both free of chemicals, and the diaper gets changed, there won't be a need for baby powder or diaper cream. You can make a cream with organic shea butter, organic lavender oil, and calendula flowers.

If you do need a cream, there is one called "Earth Mama Angel Baby Bottom Balm" that has high ratings and is safe, effective, and herbal. It is formulated with naturally antibacterial and antifungal organic herbs and oils, mineral oil, and Vitamin E, and is non-irritating and free from the most common allergens. It is also toxin-free, petroleum-free, phthalate- and paraben-free, safe for cloth diapers, lanolin- and zinc-free, and vegan! Vegan means no ingredients were derived from animals and that the products are not tested on animals, which is good for them and you.

WIPES

You will use many wipes for baby's bottom. For one baby, you can expect to go through about 2000–3000 wipes in the first year alone! Once baby gets squirmy for poopy diaper changes, you'll likely end up rinsing their tushies in the sink or bathtub.

Our skin is our largest organ, and anything we use on it goes inside of us. I preferred to have the purest wipes I could. Strangely, wipes aren't all free of chemicals, since babies' skin is so pure and sensitive. If you think about it, when we wipe our adult bottoms, we use plain toilet paper.

Did you know that store-bought baby wipes have anywhere from 10–25 ingredients?
According to the 2007 Environmental Working Group's (EWG's) analysis of hidden ingredients in cosmetics and personal care products, 95% of baby wipes are potentially contaminated with dangerous chemicals. The ingredients in store-bought baby wipes have a link to developmental problems, allergies, reproductive dysfunction, endocrine disruption, and even cancer.

FORMALDEHYDE IN DIAPER WIPES

The International Agency for Research on Cancer has defined formaldehyde as "carcinogenic to humans." According to the American Academy of Dermatology, allergic contact dermatitis is a type of eczema that develops on the skin as a result of allergic reaction. Allergic contact dermatitis usually develops a few hours after the allergen touches the skin and causes symptoms. Symptoms of exposure to formaldehyde may include:
- Itchy, swollen, and red skin or dry, bumpy skin
- Blisters may develop if the reaction is more severe
- Blisters may break, leaving crusts and scales
- Skin may later flake and crack
- With long-term exposure the skin becomes thick, red, and scaly
- Over time, the skin can darken and become leathery

Formaldehyde is a powerful chemical, and a concentration of 30 parts per million is enough to evoke an allergic reaction. Some formaldehyde-releasing preservatives release a higher amount. If you are trying to avoid formaldehyde, know that you won't find it listed as an ingredient. Instead, look for these formaldehyde-releasing preservatives:

- Diazolidinyl Urea
- DMDM Hydantoin
- Imidazolidinyl Urea
- Quaternium-15
- Tosylamide/Formaldehyde Resin
- Benzylhemiformal
- Sodium Hydroxymethylglycinate
- 2-Bromo-2-Nitropropane-1, 3-Diol (Bronopol)
- Polyoxymethylene Urea
- 5-Bromo-5-Nitro-1, 3 Dioxane
- Methenamine
- Glyoxa

∽

Avoid anything scented, since "fragrance" or "parfum" almost always means pthlalates (known endocrine disruptors). Additionally, many conventional wipes contain parabens, and some include phenoxyethanol, a suspected carcinogen. In particular, "natural" or "organic" wipes might contain phenoxyethanol as a preservative. In addition to the ingredients listed on the side of the package, there are many other chemicals that are contaminants and byproducts of the production process. These chemicals include: methylparaben, polysorbate-20, tocopheryl acetate, maleic acid, potassium laureth phosphate, tetrasodium edta, Ethylene Oxide and 1, 4-Dioxane, Hydroquinone, Bis-PEG/PPG-16/16 PEG/PPG-16/16 Dimethicone, Potassium Laureth Phosphate, Polysorbate 20, PEG-75 Lanolin, Ceteareth-20.

Sample ingredient list from mainstream supplier of "natural" wipes: water, citric acid, PEG-40 hydrogenated castor oil, benzyl alcohol, phenoxyethanol, sodium citrate, sodium benzoate, xanthan gum, disodium EDTA, BIS-PEG/PPG-16/16 PEG/PPG-16/16 dimethicone, caprylic/capric triglyceride, ethylhexylglycerin, bisabolol, chamomilla recutita (matricaria) flower extract, aloe barbadensis leaf juice

∽

I feel like if you cannot pronounce the words well, it's a great sign to not put it on the baby's body!

You can use a soft washcloth with water when at home and disposables when out and about. Look for the purest you can find, including brands like

Water Wipes, which are 99% water and 1% grapefruit seed extract. Their ingredients are as follows: purified water, citris grandis (grapefruit) seed extract, and benzalkonium chloride (trace amount).

INFANT CAR SEAT

Most hold baby until they are 30 pounds in weight, but may get too small before they weigh that much. We bought our virtually brand-new Graco at a local consignment store. We bought an extra base online so that we could have one for each car, for quick and easy car seat transferring. Popular brands of seats include Graco, Chicco, Evenflo, & Baby Trend.

STROLLER

A stroller is essential. I didn't put my son in a stroller until six months, as I loved carrying him on my body. New strollers run anywhere from $30 to $800. There is a choice between a jogging stroller with one wheel in the front or a standard 4-wheeled one. There are also "Travel Systems" with a car seat/stroller combo. Some moms may want both a standard and a jogger. They serve different purposes. But if you only get one, and want to jog, then go with a jogging one. The B.O.B. is an expensive jogging stroller, but if you get a hand-me-down or a used one, it is advantageous and adaptable. It travels well through sand, stays steady, has a good amount of pockets, and is sturdy.

The Snap-and-Go is a stroller that you can click your car seat into. Suffice it to say; there are many strollers out there. There is even one that folds up to fit in your purse! Consignment stores usually have at least 3 or 4 strollers outside the store. Make sure to test the wheels and give it a good cleaning.

BABY MONITORS

The amount of spending on baby products in the U.S. is in the billions. You and baby don't need every gadget and fancy toy. For thousands of years, there were no audio or video baby monitors. Baby monitors are one of the highest radiation emitting devices in the home, akin to a microwave. What makes baby monitors particularly dangerous is that they emit radiation full blast constantly whenever they are on. A cell phone at least only emits at full blast when sending or receiving a call.

Many of these monitors emit constant radiation 24 hours a day and are put right next to a baby. A critical study in 1996 confirmed that children are exposed to higher levels of radiation from devices than adults. Children's skulls are thinner, and ears are smaller, so radiation has a shorter distance to travel before it penetrates their brain. There are hundreds of scientific studies showing links between radio frequency radiation and crib death, cancer, DNA damage (especially in infants and fetuses) and male infertility. The World Health Organization has listed this radiation a possible "carcinogen," which means, "cancer causing."

Suggestions for protecting children from this radiation:

- Do not use a monitor. Stay within hearing distance.
- Do not place a cellular phone near the baby.
- Co-sleep with your baby. Then they are near you, happy and safe.

The American Academy of Pediatrics has recommended since 1999, that children under 2 have no screen-time whatsoever, as a child's brain develops rapidly during these early years and the best-quality learning happens live.

TEETHING

Teething is normal. It's a developmental milestone. When teething, babies most commonly experience itchy gums, not pain. They can satisfy the itch by chewing on a cool, wet washcloth. Teething gels and tablets are not only unnecessary, but some can even be dangerous, pediatricians say. Many of these products contain benzocaine, a local anesthetic. The FDA recommends against the use of benzocaine in children under two (except under the advice and supervision of a health-care professional) due to a rare, serious, sometimes fatal reaction that leads to a big reduction of oxygen in the bloodstream.

CRIBS/BASSINETS, CO-SLEEPING, BED-SHARING

Co-sleeping essentially means sleeping close to your child. It may be in the same bed or the same room. Around the globe (southern Europe, Asia, Africa, and Central and South America) to the majority of mothers and babies, co-sleeping is an unquestioned practice. Japanese parents (or grandparents) often sleep in proximity with their children until they are teenagers, referring to this arrangement as a river - the mother is one bank, the father another, and the child sleeping between them is the water. Most of the present world cultures practice a variety of co-sleeping ways, and it would never be thought acceptable or desirable to have babies sleeping alone.

In Latin America, Philippines, and Vietnam, parents sleep with their baby in a hammock next to the bed, or they place the baby in a wicker basket in the bed, between them. In Japan, many parents sleep next to their baby on bamboo or straw mats, or futons. Some put the baby in a crib or bassinet within arm's reach of the bed. Most cultures that routinely practice co-sleeping, in any form, have scarce instances of Sudden Infant Death Syndrome (SIDS). SIDS occurrences are among the lowest in the world in Hong Kong, where co-sleeping is extremely common.

According to research, from an article by James J. McKenna, Ph.D, co-sleeping is more common in the U.S. than most people believe. The typical American home has a room that contains a crib for the baby, and parents report that the baby sleeps in the crib. Yet when researchers ask specific questions about who sleeps where it turns out that the majority of mothers sleep with their young children at least some of most nights. Parents present themselves as having babies who sleep alone, following the societal norm of the baby in the baby's room and the couple in the master bedroom.

DIFFERENT WAYS OF CO-SLEEPING VARIOUS FAMILIES MAY CHOOSE

- **Bed-sharing:** The child sleeps in the same bed with the parents.
- **Sidecar:** Three sides of the crib are intact, but the side next to the parents' bed is removed or lowered, so the mother and baby have easy access to one another. Commercial co-sleeper/sidecar cribs are also available.
- **Different beds in the same room:** This might include having baby's bassinet or crib within arm reach of the parents (easier at night) or just in the same room; or preparing a pallet or bed for an older child on the floor next to, or at the foot of, the parents' bed.
- **Child welcomed into bed:** The baby/child has her own bedroom, and may start their overnight hours there, but is welcomed into the parents' bed at any time. Co-sleeping can have many advantages: Parents and babies are likely to get more sleep. Breastfeeding during the night is easier when baby is nearby, and helps to maintain milk supply. Baby stirs

and almost wakes when she needs to eat, but since she is right beside mom, mom can breastfeed or soothe her back to sleep before she fully wakes up. No nighttime separation anxiety, fewer bedtime hassles, mom doesn't have to get up and walk back and forth to another room.

Those who are uncomfortable with the idea of co-sleeping often suggest that co-sleeping is "less healthy" than the child sleeping alone and will cause psychological damage to the child, or cause the baby to become too dependent on the parents. Or they think it will ruin the parent's sex life. My aunt, when I told her that my son still slept with us at age 3, said, "Can I ask you a personal question? Where do you guys have sex then?" I assured her that there are many other places in our house to do so, other than our bed.

It has never been proven or shown, nor is it even probable that sleeping with your baby has any detrimental long-term effects when the relationships between those involved are healthy. Co-sleeping helps develop positive qualities, such as more comfort with physical affection, more confidence in one's own sexual gender identity, a more positive and optimistic attitude about life, more innovativeness as a toddler, and an increased ability to be alone. It's beautiful and joyous to sleep and wake up with your smiling baby/children!

SUDDEN INFANT DEATH SYNDROME (SIDS)

Also known as "crib death," is the sudden, unexpected death of an infant under one year of age that remains unexplained after a complete investigation, including an autopsy, examination of the death scene, and review of medical history. Approximately 2,500 babies in the U.S. die every year while sleeping, with most deaths occurring between 2–4 months of age.

Sleeping in the same room as your baby reduces the risk of Sudden Infant Death Syndrome (SIDS) by as much as 50% [American Academy of Pediatrics]. The Infant Sleep Information Source website notes: "The most recent studies have shown that most bed-sharing deaths happen when an adult sleeping with a baby has been smoking, drinking alcohol, or taking drugs (illegal or over-the-counter medicines) that make them sleep deeply." Sometimes people fall asleep with their babies accidentally or without meaning to, which can be very dangerous, especially if it happens on a couch/sofa where a baby can get wedged or trapped between the adult and the cushions.

James J. McKenna, Ph.D., a world-recognized infant sleep authority, notes:

> "Overwhelmingly, bed-sharing deaths are associated with at least one independent risk factor associated with an infant dying. These include an infant being placed prone (on its stomach) and placed in an adult bed without supervision, or no breastfeeding, or other children in the bed, or infants being placed in an adult bed on top of a pillow, or who bedshare even though their mothers smoked during the pregnancy therein compromising potentially the infants ability to arouse (to terminate too little oxygen, or to terminate an apnea). Drug use and alcohol have historically been associated with poor outcomes for bed-sharing babies, so if drugs and/or alcohol are present, please don't bed-share."

Other potential concerns in bed-sharing: very long hair should be tied up so that it does not become wrapped around baby's neck; a parent who is an exceptionally deep sleeper or an extremely obese parent who has a problem feeling exactly how close baby is should consider having a baby sleep nearby on a separate surface instead; do not swaddle baby as they may overheat and are not able to effectively move covers from the face or use arms and legs to alert an adult who is too close.

MAKE ANY AND ALL SLEEP SURFACES SAFE FOR BABY: (including bassinets, cribs, nap surfaces, or beds)

- Baby should be placed on their back to sleep.
- The sleep surface must be firm. Do not put a baby on a waterbed mattress, pillow, beanbag, sheepskin, or any other soft surface to sleep.
- The mattress should be tight fitting to the headboard and footboard (or sides of the crib). Bedding should be tight fitting to the mattress.
- There should not be loose pillows, stuffed animals, or soft blankets near the baby's face. There should not be any space between the bed and adjoining wall where the baby could roll and become trapped.
- Babies (with or without an adult) should never sleep on a sofa, couch, futon, recliner, or other surface where they can slip into a crevice or become wedged against the back of the chair/sofa/etc.

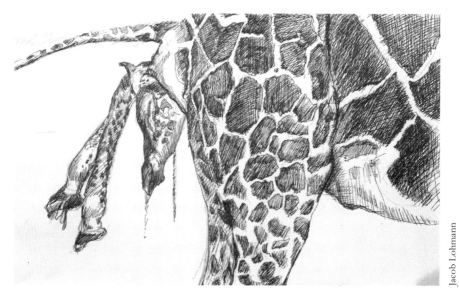

EPILOGUE

"Women's bodies have near-perfect knowledge of childbirth; it's when their brains get involved that things can go wrong."
- PEGGY VINCENT, *Baby Catcher*

WE HAVE DISTANCED OURSELVES from the fact that we are animals. We identify as humans, but we are mammals, and we are animated. The word "mammal" is from the scientific "mammalia," derived from the Latin "mamma."

When pregnant with my son, I watched videos of a dolphin, giraffe, elephant, and primate give birth. It was inspiring and instinctive. We must follow those instincts that we and all other animals have, that natural ability to be attracted to another being, to have intercourse, to reproduce, to labor, to birth, to parent. Birth is natural. Nowadays, someone says they had a "natural" birth, to distinguish that it was unmedicated. It isn't the other way around; where someone specifies with, I had a "medicated" birth. The natural birth is the one that is identified as a special case. Just as ways of life that are natural and preventative are referred to as "alternatives" to the norm.

Especially in the current climate, parents must take the initiative and fervor to educate themselves on pregnancy, labor, and birth. Generations can learn both what to do and what NOT to do from those that come before. The purpose for passion about systemic change is to flush out the root toxicity and reveal the truth. When truth comes into our culture, we can make different decisions; decisions that cause less suffering.

I humbly request that you share this book, whether it is the actual copy in your hands, or one specially purchased for someone you know. Give one to an entire high school class, your daughter, your friend's daughter, your neighbor who is expecting, a cousin, a first-time father, your granddaughter, to a pregnant mother at your church, the grocery store, or park. Place one in a "Little Free Library" down the road, buy one for a local library, donate one to a jail, or give them as college graduation gifts. Let knowledge spread like wildfires. Let superficiality become uninteresting. Let us be curious, and care for the happiness, freedom, health and well being of all beings everywhere, especially mothers and the new souls arriving to this realm.

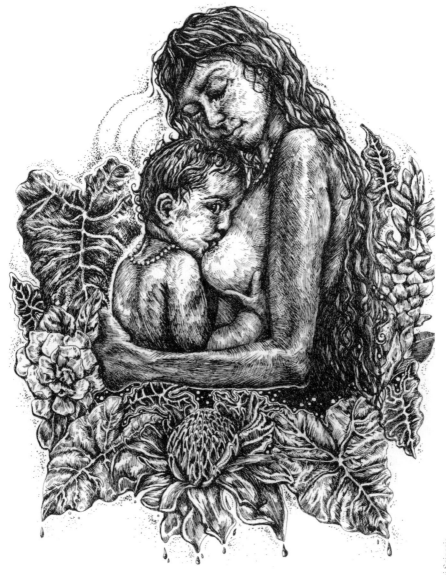

Nikki Scioscia

APPENDIX A: EXTRAS

BLESSING WAY CELEBRATION

At one point in time, women would gather together to empower and support one another as they stepped into the role of bearing and raising children. This rite of passage into motherhood was tribe life, deeply ingrained, and passed down from culture to culture, generation to generation, and woman to woman. In Native American tradition (Dine Navajo to be accurate), a ceremony called a Blessingway created space to come together as a support circle for the expecting mother, and bless the way ahead for her. It is a web woven of the most trusted and cherished women in her life.

Before baby comes, everyone gathers to bless the baby and celebrate the parents and child. A Blessingway is a great opportunity to include the father/partner. They, too, get to have people offer them advice, love, support, and shower them with the joyfulness and excitement of having a child. I felt it was such a beautiful experience, having had a baby shower with all of my closest girlfriends, sister, and mother, to then watch my husband receive everyone's attention, praise, and love, alongside me.

A Blessingway can include things such as: reading poems, playing and singing songs, offering blessings, creating a necklace of beads with beads that people chose, brought and blessed, sharing food, lighting candles, etc.

PARENTS WORKING ON THEIR CONSCIOUSNESS

When parents work on themselves, putting effort into their awareness and evolution of both their consciousness and conscious action, it can effect the population. Because beliefs and behavior are two different things and the goal is that they match up...an example of this would be something such as saying we love animals, but then contributing to killing them and then eating their body parts, and not recognizing the connection. Connection and compassion are two things that conscious parents can continue working on.

"ON CHILDREN"

The famous Lebanese artist, philosopher, and writer Kahlil Gibran lived from 1883–1931. His works, written in both Arabic and English, are full of lyrical outpourings and express our deep mystical nature. "The Prophet" is a book of 26 poetic essays, originally published in 1923, translated into over forty different languages. Below is his essay titled "On Children."

> Your children are not your children.
> They are the sons and daughters of Life's longing for itself.
> They come through you but not from you,
> And though they are with you, yet they belong not to you.
> You may give them your love but not your thoughts.
> For they have their own thoughts.
> You may house their bodies but not their souls,
> For their souls dwell in the house of tomorrow,
> which you cannot visit, not even in your dreams.
> You may strive to be like them, but seek not to make them like you.
> For life goes not backward nor tarries with yesterday.
> You are the bows from which your children as living arrows are
>   sent forth.
> The archer sees the mark upon the path of the infinite,
> and He bends you with His might that His arrows may go swift
>   and far.
> Let your bending in the archer's hand be for gladness;
> For even as He loves the arrow that flies,
> so He loves also the bow that is stable.

MEDITATION

Meditating can be a very useful practice, not only for parents, but for everyone. Some benefits of meditating are patience, poise, acceptance, equanimity, ability to watch the mind without identifying with it, ability to focus in the present moment, ability to be still inward and out, forgiveness of oneself, forgiveness of others, knowing the habit patterns of mind, knowing the true nature of the mind, lowered blood pressure, etc.

STAY IN THE PRESENT MOMENT & AVOID LIKE/DISLIKE

One thing that children help us with is being in the present moment. Often, we pull them out of it by asking them about the past and future. Also do your best not to reinforce "like and dislike" "good and bad" etc. miring them into a world of preference. Let them develop and explore without prejudice as best you can. Try not to reinforce these constant words of division.

This is an excerpt from a book I found in a small bookstore in Australia called *Ridding Yourself of Unhappiness* by Barry Long:

> "The child is continuously exposed to conversations like this:
>
> "Did you have a good (exciting or get-what-you-like) time on the holiday you were looking forward (for excitement) to?"
>
> "Yes, it was interesting (not so exciting) but it was very depressing (negatively exciting) when…How have you been?"
>
> "We've been well (meaning physically, no mention of love of the beauty or truth of life) but John is unhappy (negatively excited) about his job. He had a wonderful (exciting) promotion but…"
>
> "What did you do yesterday?" (the questioner is looking for excitement, not love or life.)
>
> "Nothing much (no excitement). But tonight we're having a dinner party (excitement to look forward to, and more conversations like this one about likes and dislikes."
>
> Apart from the influence of their friends, the parent's attachment to their false and unhappy selves—possessing physic identity—is kept alive and vibrant for them by society's relentless stimulation of their likes and dislikes."

LOKAH SAMASTAH SUKHINO BHAVANTU

This is a mantra that means may all beings in this location of the universe be happy, sweet, joyful, centered, and free as we are meant to be. May all we think, say, and do contribute to the happiness and freedom for everyone.

LULLABY

May the longtime sun, shine upon you, all love-surround you, and the pure light within you, guide your way on.

RESPECT THEIR MIND/HEART/VOICE

Avoid controlling your children, never respecting that they too have an opinion, desires, and feelings. Respect their voice. Their desires are important. If children always feel controlled, they will lose a sense of empowerment. Giving them options and choices, hearing what they have to say is essential. Why do adults think they can be moody, crabby, and change their mind, but children cannot?

For several months, my child didn't want to get in his car seat, so it was a struggle. I was full of hormones, tired, and frustrated. If I wanted to leave the grocery store or had to be somewhere, I would try to coerce him and then physically force him into his seat. It didn't feel good to he or I. So I went online one night to a website called The Natural Child Project, where I found helpful information. The next day, when he didn't want to get into his seat, I had a new tool I had read of. This time, I responded to him by saying, "Okay. Let me know when you are ready." He calmed down and about two minutes later, climbed into his seat. I could feel a shift in both him and myself that informs me to this day.

INCLUDE THEM & UNDERSTAND THEM

Often when adults are together, telling a story or talking to each other, they may look at everyone around the table or room, but never at the child (or children). The child is there too. Make eye contact with them. Include them in the conversation. This inclusiveness is an expression of respect for their hearts and minds and presence.

If you are walking with a child, urging them to "hurry up," keep in mind that an adult's legs are much longer than those of a child. Give them time to walk at a pace they can. They will not be able to walk as fast as you. They are never in a hurry, because they live in the present moment.

It is so important to be a child. Allow them to be little, remember how small they are. Saying things like, "Oh you're so big. Such a big girl," can lead to them thinking they need to be "big," and not who they are.

Sometimes when children lose things or break something, a big deal is made out of it, but if an adult loses their keys or drops a glass and it breaks, it's fine and normal.

HOW TO REALLY LOVE A CHILD

by Susan Ariel Rainbow Kennedy (SARK bestselling author & artist PlanetSARK.com)

Be there.

Say yes as often as possible.

Let them bang on pots and pans.

If they're unlovable, love them.

Realize how important it is to be a child.

Go to a movie theatre in your pajamas.

Read books out loud with joy.

Play together.

Remember how really small they are.

Giggle a lot.

Surprise them.

Say no when necessary.

Teach feelings.

Let God heal your own inner child.

Learn about parenting.

Hug trees together.

Make loving safe.

Bake a cake and eat it with no hands.

Go find elephants and kiss them.

Plan to build a rocket ship.

Make lots of forts with blankets.

Reveal your own dreams.

Search out the positive.

Keep the gleam in your eye.

Mail letters to God.

Encourage silly.

Plant licorice in your garden.

Open up.

Stop yelling.

Express your Love—A Lot!

Speak kindly.

Paint their tennis shoes.

HANDLE WITH CARING.

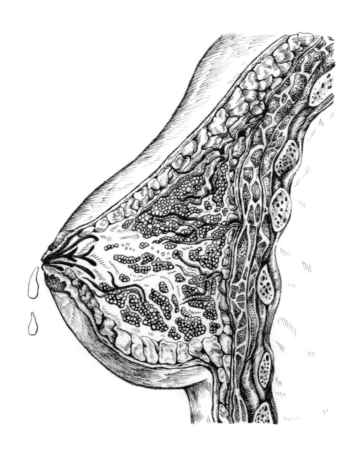

APPENDIX B: SUGGESTED BOOKS, FILMS, WEBSITES

BOOKS

Sacred Birthing by Sunni Karll

Bountiful, Beautiful, Blissful by Gurmukh Kaur Khalsa

Choices in Pregnancy and Childbirth, John Wilks

Ina May's Guide to Childbirth, Ina May Gaskin

Spiritual Midwifery by Ina May Gaskin

Birth Stories by Ina May Gaskin

Placenta, The Forgotten Chakra by Robin Lim

After the Baby's Born: A Woman's Way to Wellness: A Complete Guide for Postpartum Women, Robin Lim

Birth by Tina Cassidy

Pushed, Jennifer Block

Babies Are Not Pizzas: They're Born, Not Delivered, by Rebecca Dekker

The Parents Tao Te Cheng, translation by William Martin

The Great Mother

Hypnobirthing by Marie F Mongan

Breastfeeding without Birthing by Dr. Jack Newman

Conceiving Souls of Magnificence by Sunni Karll

The Natural Child: Parenting from the Heart by Jan Hunt

Baby Catcher by Peggy Vincent

Magical Child by Joseph Chilton Pearce

The Awakened Family by Dr. Shefali Tsabary

Conscious Parenting by Dr. Shefali Tsabary

Healer's Guide to High Vibes: Practical Ways to Cleanse Your Energy Field by Helen Greenfield

The Continuum Concept by Jean Liedloff

Gentle Birth, Gentle Mothering by Dr. Sarah J Buckley

Mama Glow: A Hip Guide to Your Fabulous Abundant Pregnancy by Latham Thomas

FILMS

Happy Healthy Child (4 part series)
Birth Story: Ina May Gaskin
American Circumcision
The Business of Being Born
Mother May I?
Microbirth

What Baby Wants
Vaxxed
Why Not Home?
All My Babies: A Midwife's Own Story
Freedom for Birth

WEBSITES

Birthmonopoly.com
Evidencebasedbirth.com
Exposingthesilenceproject.com
Humanizebirth.org
Pattch.org
Birthmatters.org
Intactamerica.org
Doctorsopposingcircumcision.org
Learntherisk.org
Restoringforeskin.org
Noharmm.org
Thenaturalchildproject.com

VBAC.com
Midwifethinking.com
Improvingbirth.org
Waterbirth.org
Sarahbuckley.com
Asklenore.info
Iblce.org
Bumisehat.org
Midwiferytoday.com
Ican-online.org
Tatia.org
Naturalchild.org